PRAISE FOR *THE DIRTY, LAZY, KETO COOKBOOK*

"Stephanie Laska's results speak for themselves. If you're ready to 'go keto' but need help along the way (and who doesn't), this book is your go-to guide."

—**Chris Guillebeau**, *New York Times* bestselling author of *Side Hustle* and *The $100 Startup*

"As a board-certified obesity medicine specialist, I endeavor to keep my finger on the pulse of current dietary and weight loss trends.… Stephanie GETS IT! It is obvious to me that she has done her homework.…She has forged for herself better health and a better life and is providing tools for others to do the same."

—**Michael W. Jones**, DO, MBA, FAAFP, medical bariatrician

"By writing *The DIRTY, LAZY, KETO Cookbook*, Stephanie and William Laska created a gem. Keto dieters rejoice! No more confusing information and no more guessing games. Expect to have fun and lose weight with this book."

—**Nordine Zouareg**, international fitness and wellness expert, former Mr. Universe, and author of *InnerFitness: 5 Steps to Eliminating Inner Conflict and Creating Inner Peace*

"Stephanie and William Laska have written a cookbook that you will find yourself using every day and is sure to be a godsend in helping you succeed on a low-carb lifestyle.…The recipes taste terrific and are simple to make. They also recognize that some of us have different needs by providing an easy-to-use categorization system that identifies things like budget-friendly or high-volume dishes. Where has this cookbook been all my life?"

—**Dr. Tamara Sniezek**, professor of sociology and cohost of the *DIRTY, LAZY, Girl* podcast

THE DIRTY, LAZY, KETO COOKBOOK

BEND THE RULES TO LOSE THE WEIGHT!

Stephanie Laska, MEd, and William Laska

ADAMS MEDIA

New York   London   Toronto   Sydney   New Delhi

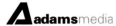

Adams Media
An Imprint of Simon & Schuster, Inc.
57 Littlefield Street
Avon, Massachusetts 02322

First Adams Media trade paperback edition January 2020

ADAMS MEDIA and colophon are trademarks of Simon & Schuster.

For information about special discounts for bulk purchases, please contact Simon & Schuster Special Sales at 1-866-506-1949 or business@ simonandschuster.com.

The Simon & Schuster Speakers Bureau can bring authors to your live event. For more information or to book an event contact the Simon & Schuster Speakers Bureau at 1-866-248-3049 or visit our website at www.simonspeakers.com.

Interior design by Colleen Cunningham
Photographs by James Stefiuk
Interior images © Getty Images/maglyvi, nadyaillyustrator, Serhii Sereda, Nadzeya_Dzivakova, petite_lili, LanaMay; 123RF/sudowoodo, macrovector, Aksana Chubis, Mikalai Manyshau
Author photographs by William Laska

Manufactured in the United States of America

10 9 8 7 6 5 4 3 2 1

Library of Congress Cataloging-in-Publication Data
Names: Laska, Stephanie, author. | Laska, William, author.
Title: The DIRTY, LAZY, KETO cookbook / Stephanie Laska, MEd, and William Laska.
Description: Avon, Massachusetts: Adams Media, 2020.
Identifiers: LCCN 2019038555 | ISBN 9781507212301 (pb) | ISBN 9781507212318 (ebook)
Subjects: LCSH: Reducing diets. | Low-carbohydrate diet--Recipes. | Ketogenic diet. | Health. | Quick and easy cooking. | LCGFT: Cookbooks.
Classification: LCC RM237.73 .L37 2020 | DDC 641.5/6383--dc23
LC record available at https://lccn.loc.gov/ 2019038555

ISBN 978-1-5072-1230-1
ISBN 978-1-5072-1231-8 (ebook)

Always follow safety and commonsense cooking protocols while using kitchen utensils, operating ovens and stoves, and handling uncooked food. If children are assisting in the preparation of any recipe, they should always be supervised by an adult.

The information in this book should not be used for diagnosing or treating any health problem. Not all diet and exercise plans suit everyone. You should always consult a trained medical professional before starting a diet, taking any form of medication, or embarking on any fitness or weight training program. The author and publisher disclaim any liability arising directly or indirectly from the use of this book.

DEDICATION

From Stephanie:

If you've been shamed by the keto police, or criticized for not following a diet plan perfectly, then this book is dedicated to you. I'm living proof that weight loss is possible without such rigid guidelines. Every time I hear, "but that's not keto," I want to say, "Oh *realllllllllly?* Could you please hold my Diet Coke (or low-carb beer!) while I zip up my size 4 skinny jeans?" Seriously, though… there is *another* way to keto, and it's healthy, effective, *and* sustainable! I started the rebellious DIRTY, LAZY, KETO book series with two guiding messages in mind:

1. You are not alone with your weight loss struggles. Many of us, including me, don't seem to have an "off switch" when it comes to carbs. That doesn't make us bad people. We just need a different approach.
2. You don't have to be perfect to be successful. Weight loss is possible without so many strict rules! There is more than one way to keto. I'm going to introduce you to mine.

I am here to support you, dear readers. From the grocery store to the kitchen table, let's bend the rules to lose the weight!

A special thanks to my husband and coauthor, who supported me and this extraordinary lifestyle change, every step of the way.

#KetoOn!

Stephanie

From William:

We have all been there. Standing in the kitchen with a cookbook in front of us with a delicious recipe chosen. But what happens next is a terrible letdown. You start reading the long list of exotic ingredients and realize you either don't know what they are, or don't have the necessary items in your kitchen. Perhaps first you see something innocent like lemon zest on the list. *Hmmm…that's not so bad.* But then, the alarm bells really start to go off when you come across an ingredient you're not 100 percent familiar with, like chives, scallions, or shallots. *"What the heck is a shallot?"* you might be thinking. If you're like me, this is where you consider slamming the cookbook shut and ordering takeout. (Note: All three are very similar to the green onion, and in this cookbook, that is what we will call it!) Why are cookbooks often so complicated? I just want to make dinner tonight without any annoying or expensive obstacles.

As the coauthor of *The DIRTY, LAZY, KETO Cookbook*, my goal was to bring forth recipes and meals that weren't overcomplicated, but still taste delicious. I wanted to support my wife as she lost 140 pounds, but in a way that wouldn't make us go broke, or crazy, trying to find ridiculous-sounding ingredients at ten different grocery stores.

Let's have fun cooking together, folks, but in a way that's straightforward and fun. I'd like to dedicate this cookbook to *those* DIRTY, LAZY, KETO peeps. Join my family in the DLK kitchen, and *let's do this together!*

Special thanks to my liveliest recipe testers, Charlotte and Alex. Thank you for your patience and understanding while Mom and Dad embark on this keto journey to spread the word of this unbelievable way of eating that has such profound potential to change and save lives!

#KetoOn!
Bill

CONTENTS

THE DIRTY, LAZY, KETO METHOD

1. BE A KETO REBEL

2. DIRTY, LAZY, KETO PREP FOR COOKING

9. DRINKS AND DESSERTS

PREFACE

When people ask, "What made you finally decide to lose the weight?" I've been known to sarcastically reply, "Well, I REALLY liked being fat!" Seriously, though: When my doctor told me that I had reached Morbid Obesity Stage III on the BMI scale, I didn't even flinch. It didn't seem real.

What I did know is that I felt severely uncomfortable in my skin—I weighed close to 300 pounds. Even though (at the time) I didn't suffer from any obvious or immediate health problems, I knew if I didn't "do something" I would likely end up with diabetes or someday be stuffed into an extra-large coffin.

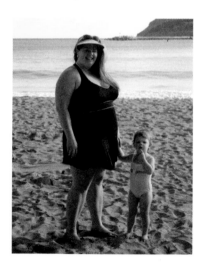 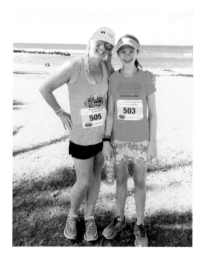

So how did I end up losing about half of my total body weight?

It wasn't until I was riding a roller coaster when it really hit home. My companion on the ride, my five-year-old son, almost flew out of the roller coaster after the first hill. Because I was so large, the pull-down bar reached only my stomach, leaving a huge, unprotected gap between it and my little boy. I spent the entire ride absolutely terrified—not because of the intended thrills—but because I was horrified that my son would fly out of the car.

People aren't fat because they are lazy or selfish; they simply *don't know* how to lose weight and keep it off. This roller coaster moment was a tipping point for me where I decided I absolutely had to figure this stuff out—like right now.

I would've done anything, absolutely anything, at that moment to get rid of my excess fat. Before resorting to weight loss surgery, which I considered being the "end of the line," I decided to try one last dietary intervention. I had heard about Atkins and keto, but both seemed too strict for me. Trying to eat "perfectly" all the time, I realized, would set me up for a lifetime of disappointment and rebellion.

Strict Keto dieters give up everything fun. Artificial sweeteners like Splenda are frowned upon by the keto police, as are fat bombs and a cold, low-carb beer. Even a scoop of low-carb ice cream is out of the question (who invited *THAT* guy to the party?). I couldn't understand how anyone could give up Diet Coke or tortillas. Let's keep it real. My limited family budget didn't include 100 percent organic vegetables, line-caught fish, or grass-fed butter. Call me crass, but at the time, most of my meals came from the microwave or a drive-thru.

According to the diet books I had read, that meant I was doomed to fail. But what if "they" were wrong? There had to be another way. The secret to my success was tossing out the established "rules" for weight loss and essentially learning to play dirty.

I learned to listen to my own physical and emotional needs, rebelling against the traditional beliefs of what healthy eating is supposed to look like.

I discovered, by accident, that by eating somewhat of a higher-fat, moderate-protein, lower-carbohydrate diet, but without restrictive rules, I could *finally* solve my weight loss riddle.

I bucked the system by proving I could lose a significant amount of weight—140 pounds!—and keep it off for *years—six years and counting!* The only catch? I had to do it my way.

The result was a kinder, more inclusive version of keto. DIRTY, LAZY, KETO is not obsessive like other Strict Keto diets, where folks count carbs from their toothpaste or multivitamin. **DIRTY, LAZY, KETO allows sugar substitutes, grain alternatives, and a more flexible method of counting macronutrients. You can have your sugar-free cake, and eat it too.** *Hallelujah!*

If you're a keto dropout who is tired of trying to be perfect (or were too intimidated even to start!), then this cookbook is for you.

You don't have to be perfect to be successful! I'm living proof that sustainable weight loss is possible *without* following unnecessary and constrictive rules. If I can lose 140 pounds by enjoying a "dirty" and "lazy" form of keto, then I'm betting you can too!

Let's do this together, my friend; let's do this in *our own way.*

INTRODUCTION

Most keto books on the market do not speak to me. I'm not sure who their audience is, but I am not a member. In my opinion, there are too many rules to follow on a strict ketogenic diet. The percentages, macro goals, and "rules" about ingredients are unnecessarily complex and laborious. It made me wonder—does it need to be so convoluted? I lost a huge amount of weight without tracking every morsel I put into my mouth. I never dissected macro ratios. I didn't have ketosis goals. I haven't found a keto cookbook yet that speaks to me, so that's why I decided to write one.

> Traditional cookbooks often read like a steamy romance novel. They're adventurous, full of exotic experiences and have a perfect ending. This is all fantasy. I don't know about you, but my pathetic efforts to make these elaborate dishes usually end in a giant belly flop.

This cookbook keeps things simple. I don't have enough gas in my tank to drive around to specialty stores or stop by a farmers' market. I operate in a small kitchen and with a tight budget, and I am still able to make simple, delicious, keto-friendly recipes. My life is busy, and honestly, I have only the time (and skills!) to make meals that are fast, easy, and inexpensive. And there's nothing wrong with that—you don't have to be rich or a professional chef to lose weight; you just need a simple plan that fits your life.

The DIRTY, LAZY, KETO Cookbook is about fixing delicious food fast and under budget.

Nothing fancy here! With this in mind, this cookbook will give you:

+ 100 stress-free recipes with simple instructions
+ Common ingredients that are easy to find (at any grocery or big-box store)
+ Low net carb recipes that fit within the DIRTY, LAZY, KETO lifestyle
+ Tips to make recipes "family-friendly"
+ Honesty—this is what I eat and make for my family

You'll also find that the recipes are divided into helpful categories:

$ **BUDGET FRIENDLY:** These recipes have inexpensive ingredients for the cost-conscious chef.

PERFECT FOR VOLUME EATERS: These recipes are for when you're extra hungry or simply like big portions (like me).

✗ **PICKY EATERS:** These favorite dishes are for even the most discerning palates, both young and old.

◎ **FANCY ENOUGH FOR GUESTS:** These dishes are great to share at special events.

VEGETARIAN-"ISH": These recipes do not contain meat, but may contain dairy and eggs.

KETO SUPERSTARS: These dishes are trusted keto favorites.

I also don't plan on sending you out into the kitchen all alone. This is a full-service experience! In *The DIRTY, LAZY, KETO Cookbook* you will also find my weekly grocery list of recommended foods to keep on hand. I will suggest sugar and starch alternatives and tricks to incorporate more vegetables into your diet.

What is the difference between a chive, a green onion, and a scallion? Sorry for putting you on the spot, but I don't know either. If I don't know what an ingredient is, it doesn't belong in my cookbook.

The goal of this easy cookbook is to help you put theory into practice. *The DIRTY, LAZY, KETO Cookbook* opens my vault of recipes that helped me to lose weight. They are unique, but not complicated. You will instantly recognize some traditional family favorites, while others take on a completely fresh approach. I still enjoy these recipes to maintain my weight loss.

It's an honor and a privilege to pass along my knowledge to you.

THE DIRTY, LAZY, KETO METHOD

One Carb at a Time

CHAPTER 1

BE A KETO REBEL

Dirty Keto—I swear it's not X-rated. Dirty Keto isn't X-rated, but the phrase is often whispered in the dark corners of anonymous keto chat rooms. Rules are being broken with Dirty Keto, and dieters are made to feel ashamed.

I don't know about you, but I've been trying to follow society's norms about dieting for my entire life; sadly, even when I followed the "rules" of healthy eating, I just couldn't lose weight. I ate oatmeal for breakfast like my doctor told me to do, and I substituted natural honey for sugar. I chose whole grains for my breads and pastas. I drank smoothies and skim milk, snacked on fruit to keep me full, and purchased fat-free crackers and snacks. I never used butter, and I passed on fattening foods like eggs, mayo, and nuts. Despite following all of these "rules," my weight spiraled out of control. *That's just not fair.*

Hovering close to 300 pounds, I spent my adult life avoiding booths at restaurants and passing up amusement park rides fearing I wouldn't fit behind the safety bar. I once placed a jacket over my lap and pretended to be asleep, praying the flight attendant wouldn't notice that my seatbelt *could not close.*

I've tried so many diets, but none of them had any positive, lasting results. The calorie-restrictive model of weight loss actually caused me to *gain weight, not lose weight.* I felt constantly hungry and resentful about not being able to enjoy my favorite foods. Like a hunter, I would search for ways to skirt the system. I remember being on the Weight Watcher's Fat and Fiber plan (many years ago) where foods were awarded a point value based on their "health content" *or something equally subjective*. I discovered a delicious bran muffin at Trader Joe's that miraculously ranked low in points. I wish I had bought stock in that grocery store chain because I bought and ate those muffins by the pallet! I even became somewhat of a muffin dealer at my weekly support meeting, selling four-packs out of the trunk of my car *for a slight profit*. Every single one of us stayed within our "point range" while eating those "healthy" muffins, but predictably, we all gained weight.

I have a hard time following rules that don't make sense. The trendy keto diet is no different from other formal dieting plans in that there are precise rules to follow. Keto's strict prescription for weight loss is clear: Eat no more than 20 grams of carbs per day to lose weight—no exceptions. Calories must be distributed by a perfect ratio of 75 percent fat, 20 percent protein, and 5 percent carbohydrate. If a secret handbook existed for Strict Keto dieters, hypothetically, this is what it might say:

1. Eat only "whole" foods grown above the ground.
2. Do not eat precooked or prepackaged foods.
3. Prepare your own meals.
4. Do not eat foods with chemicals or unnatural ingredients.

Wow! I wouldn't last a day in that club. I'm confident the strict ketogenic diet is effective when followed to a T; ketosis leads to weight loss. The scientific principles behind the ketogenic diet are indeed spot on.

I also agree with the science behind the keto diet, but not its current police state implementation. Life is complicated; people like me need some breathing room in order to be successful. I'm not going to lose weight by tracking numbers in a calculator— that's just not my style. I also like drinking Diet Coke and *maybe even a beer*—does that mean I can't "do keto"? Let's get serious, people. There has to be another way that doesn't require you counting carbs from your toothpaste and multivitamin.

I've been criticized and laughed at for my vision of DIRTY, LAZY, KETO; at times, I've been made to feel that I've even done something wrong. But in the end, when I hop on a scale, I see my weight has literally been cut by 50 percent from where I started.

Can I suggest something crazy here that maybe no one else has thought of yet—*maybe my way works too*?

Dirty Keto might feel devious or subversive to some, but I call it liberating. There is room for all of us on the keto bandwagon, no matter our unique methods. We don't all have to follow the same set of rules; let's lose weight *a la keto–style* by following slightly different paths to reach the same goal.

DIRTY, LAZY, KETO is flexible and sustainable. Because I'm not holding myself up to some impossible standard of perfection, I'm less likely to throw in the towel after making a mistake. I forgive myself, then jump right back in. It's flexible too. The way I look at food has completely changed. At social events, instead of staring at my phone to calculate macro percentages, I feel relaxed and confident about what I choose to eat. Instead of being stressed about how vacations, birthdays, and weekends will impact my eating, I feel armed with strategies and tools for weight loss success. DIRTY, LAZY, KETO is so accommodating that it has become my way of life. *I can, and will, eat this way forever.*

It's not just my attitude about keto that makes me dirty. *Dirty Keto* also references my open-door policy toward substituting ingredients. For example, instead of cane sugar, Dirty Keto dieters use sugar substitutes like Splenda. In place of white flour, almond flour. The type of sugar and flour substitutes you choose is a matter of personal choice or preference. Available options are often artificially made or chemically processed during manufacturing, and for some reason, this issue provokes absolute rage among Strict Keto dieters.

There is no judgment here, my friends! While some keto authors criticize your decision to include artificial or processed sugars/flours in your diet, here it is encouraged.

It has been my experience that cooking with these "culinary crutches" makes recipes taste more "like you are used to" and therefore more enjoyable. I would even go so far as to say that sugar and flour substitutes make it possible for DIRTY, LAZY, KETO to be sustainable over the long haul. I no longer "miss out" on foods I previously enjoyed. A DIRTY, LAZY, KETO substitute or close alternative *always* exists.

Am I trading one problem for another by eating artificial sugars in my diet? (Probably!) But hey, I'm going to pick my poison here. On any given day, I feel I am one trip to the vending machine away from gaining all of my weight back. If having a piece of sugar-free candy prevents me from "falling off the wagon" so to speak, then count me in!

> What's more dangerous to my health—enduring complications of morbid obesity or drinking Splenda-sweetened coffee?

The nutrition police are out in droves right now screaming, "BUT THAT'S NOT KETO!" Don't worry, my friends. Relax and enjoy your Diet Coke or drink your low-carb beer. I am fighting back on your behalf (while wearing my size 4 skinny jeans!).

Additionally, I interpret *Dirty Keto* to include a no-holds-barred approach to dieting. As the creator of DIRTY, LAZY, KETO, I like to break the rules every once in a while. Flexibility is the key differentiator here, making this a realistic lifestyle.

LAZY KETO—DON'T SWEAT THE SMALL STUFF

Lazy Keto doesn't mean resting on the couch. Typically, Lazy Keto dieters "count" only net carbs. *Lazy Keto* is an expression for monitoring only net carbs (not fat, protein, or calories).

For me, Lazy Keto also means I mentally tally how many carbs I eat every day without the use of a formal tracking system. Not everyone can get away with this, I understand. Because I'm a rebel, using a more formal accountability system would cause me more harm than good. If I had to write down everything that I ate in a tracker, I would tell lies and omit dalliances—*to myself of all people!*

Even popular mobile apps lead me to rebel. I admit how immature that all sounds, but it's my truth.

> *Work with* your personality, *not against it* to monitor your eating habits.

Some people thrive with accountability. I have a friend at work that gets so much joy out of documenting her food choices. I think it's reassuring for her to plug in every morsel she eats into an online diary. My colleague makes better eating choices knowing that what she eats is being tabulated—it allows her to stop obsessing over what to eat next. The tracker is motivating and helpful for her, not demoralizing or cumbersome. She is using an effective strategy based on her personality type. That's a win! To achieve success with this approach, a person has to be honest and consistent, and when tracking the minutiae of my diet, I'm neither. My coworker diligently documents her accurate food intake like it's a homework assignment; I'm betting she will succeed! Whether your personality type is more aligned to that of my tracking friend, or more rebellious like me, capitalize on and harness your personal tendencies to achieve the desired outcome. Don't try to be someone else. Do what works for you, I say, and your results will improve.

> Please, for the love of all things keto, don't try to change who you are. DO WHAT WORKS FOR YOU.

HOW DIRTY, LAZY, KETO IS DIFFERENT

If you haven't guessed already, I am the poster child for the DIRTY, LAZY, KETO method. I eat between 20 and 50 grams of net carbs per day. That's quite a big range, people! Some days (or weeks) I eat toward the lower end of the range (20 grams of net carbs), and other days, I push the limits (50 grams of net carbs). Why is that? Was this part of a calculated nutritional plan? *Nope!* Trial and error, remember? While I was losing 140 pounds, I did not have a map for what the future looked like. To be honest, I constantly worried my winning streak would end and expected the magic to wear off!

Seriously, though: I chose to eat within *a range of net carbs* as opposed to a set limit because a range allows for real life to happen. Having a little wiggle room gives me power to overcome roadblocks, challenges, and dips in my motivation. Ironically, by giving myself some freedom, I created a flexible environment where I could still be successful. I lost weight. It was freaking magical!

This is the part in the story where most readers start to wonder, "HOW LONG DID IT TAKE?"

While I may have said all of this in the beginning, it doesn't hurt to remind you again, my dear reader, THAT THIS REALLY WORKS. I lost around 10 pounds a month, *steadily*, for about a year and a half. I lost 140 pounds altogether. *I literally lost half of my entire body.*

The weirdest part, I admit (I don't want to jinx myself here), was that *it wasn't that hard.* Please don't slam the book shut at this point and run screaming from the room yelling, "This girl is CRAAAAAAAZY!" I'm being serious. Once I figured out what I was doing (like how to read a nutrition label), the whole thing just flowed for me. Yes, there were obstacles along the way, but looking at the big picture here…I quickly realized that DIRTY, LAZY, KETO was a way I could really eat, *like forever*, and be happy! I'm betting *you can do this too with the same success.*

Will a 20g to 50g range of net carbs work *exactly the same* for you? Maybe, but maybe not. I wish there was a one-size-fits-all solution. That would be so simple! Unfortunately, an easy solution like that doesn't exist. There are other factors that influence how many carbs are right for you: Age, body build, gender, hormones, and activity level all affect your metabolism. You will have to do a little experimenting of your own. Try starting with a range that makes sense to you, and see what happens!

The dramatic improvement in my overall health—not just with weight loss—compels me to share my story.

If I can help even one person climb out of the carbohydrate-laden hole that they have dug themselves into, out from the horrible cycle of feeling like crap all the time, then this will all have been worth it. (Sorry, starting to well up a bit here.)

10 GRAMS OF NET CARBS OR LESS? KEEPIN' IT REAL

This morning I stumbled upon a popular keto website boasting an assortment of keto dessert recipes. Like any carb addict, I immediately clicked on the brownie recipe. My mouth was watering until I read the macronutrients—20g carbs per serving. TWENTY! First of all, who eats just one brownie? I generally eat at least three servings of batter by licking the spoon before the pan even hits the oven. Based on some rough calculations, that brownie recipe could potentially eat up all of my carb budget for days—NO THANK YOU! Even without all of my spatula licking, 20g carbs for one serving of, well, *anything* seems way too high for my liking. Yes, I believe you can spend your daily carbs however you want, but in my experience, spending them all at once on a single keto brownie probably won't work out well for the rest of the day.

In order to keep my blood sugar stable and prevent overeating, I operate by an unspoken rule: *10 grams of net carbs or less.* If a serving of food has more than 10g net carbs per serving, *pass*! This simple strategy helped me to lose eleven sizes in clothes.

The DIRTY, LAZY, KETO Cookbook contains a hundred recipes for breakfast, lunch, dinner, snacks, drinks, and let's not forget—desserts!—all of which contain, you guessed it, less than 10g net carbs. To keep this cookbook simple, the calculated amount of net carbs per serving in the recipe is called out. I want meal planning to be as easy as possible for you! Remember, DIRTY, LAZY, KETO shouldn't be complicated.

HOW TO CALCULATE NET CARBS ON DIRTY, LAZY, KETO

To calculate your net carbs, you'll need to know how to read a nutrition label. Here is an example:

1. Notice the serving size.
2. Find the Total Carbohydrate number.
3. Subtract the amount of Dietary Fiber.
4. Subtract the amount of Sugar Alcohol (if applicable).
5. The result is the NET CARBS per serving.

Nutrition Facts

Serving Size 1/2 Cup (64g)
Servings Per Container 4

Amount Per Serving

Calories 80	Calories from Fat 25

	% Daily Values*
Total Fat 2.5g	4%
Saturated Fat 1.5g	8%
Trans Fat 0g	
Cholesterol 45mg	15%
Sodium 110mg	5%
Total Carbohydrate 13g	4%
Dietary Fiber 2g	8%
Sugars 6g	
Sugar Alcohol 5g	
Protein 5g	10%
Vitamin A 2%	Vitamin C 0%
Calcium 10%	Iron 2%

*Percent Daily Values are based on a 2,000 calorie diet.

13
−2
−5
(6)

AVOID

Bread

Pasta

Sugar

Milk

Corn

Beans

Rice

THE DIRTY, LAZY, KETO FOOD PYRAMID

Use the pyramid as a recommendation for how to spend your daily net carbs.

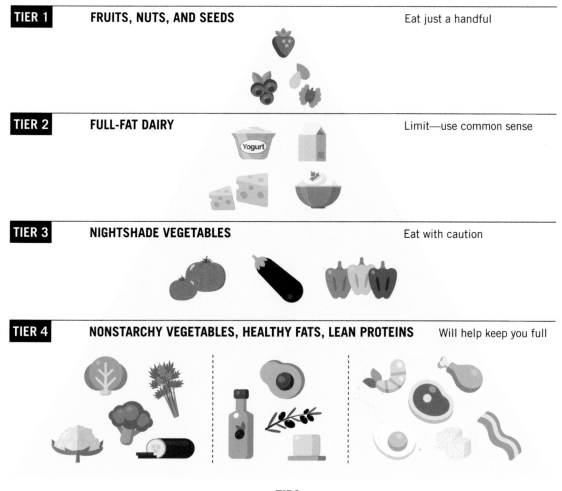

TIER 1 **FRUITS, NUTS, AND SEEDS** Eat just a handful

TIER 2 **FULL-FAT DAIRY** Limit—use common sense

TIER 3 **NIGHTSHADE VEGETABLES** Eat with caution

TIER 4 **NONSTARCHY VEGETABLES, HEALTHY FATS, LEAN PROTEINS** Will help keep you full

TIPS
Eat lots of nonstarchy vegetables!
Eat fats with your vegetables to make them more enjoyable.
Use fat only for satiety and satisfaction, not as a goal or as a food group.

DRINKS

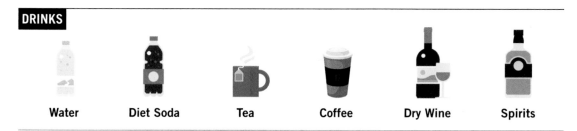

Water Diet Soda Tea Coffee Dry Wine Spirits

CHAPTER 2

DIRTY, LAZY, KETO PREP FOR COOKING

Why should you listen to me? I grew up in the Midwest, where Jell-O with Cool Whip was considered to be a salad. My childhood diet consisted of processed foods with their own jingles on TV. My preferred snacks came from a box, not a farm. To this day, I'm still haunted by the smells of sizzling Steak-umms! Looking back, I realize I completely lacked knowledge about nutrition—I believed popcorn was a vegetable since it came from corn—*seriously*.

My culinary résumé is best described as "boots on the ground," combat-style learning. There have been fires and explosions along the way, but they all led to victorious weight loss results. However quirky my recipes seem, eating these foods helped me to lose 140 pounds and maintain that weight loss for six years! That's longer than all of high school or even a presidential term.

What I lack in formal training is made up for with heart, honesty, and humor. Did I invent all of these recipes? Absolutely not! There is a quiet army of DIRTY, LAZY, KETO eaters who swap, share, and modify popular low-carb recipes. I have collected and tweaked these recipes to meet the needs of my family, budget, and personal preferences. I encourage you to do the same.

Take my ideas here and make them your own.
That's the key to success!

Throughout the cookbook, I will also be providing amusing commentary (would you expect anything less?) as we make this journey together. I will talk to you as if you were my best friend and shower you with unsolicited advice. My goal is to inspire and empower you. DIRTY, LAZY, KETO doesn't have to be complicated! This will not be a traditional cookbook experience. You might even find some of my recipes to be downright strange. Have I piqued your curiosity?

THERE ARE NO SHORTCUTS

Not everyone shares a passion for cooking. Some folks would rather turn to a meal replacement shake for a quick fix. I understand the temptation to take a shortcut—don't get me wrong! But hear me out: A shake is not a long-term solution. What happens when you stop drinking the shake? *Exactly.*

Similarly, I am weary of structured meal plans that supposedly guarantee weight loss. I wish there was a magic instruction manual to help all of us change our eating habits with a standardized plan, but sadly, you and I both know that doesn't exist. Why don't prescribed meal plans work? Because there is no "one-size-fits-all" weight loss solution. Your body is unique. Your starting weight and activity level differ greatly from the person next to you. To complicate things further, age, medication, and health conditions affect your ability to lose weight.

Personalized weight loss is the key to success. Once you figure out which guidelines work for you, I suspect you are more likely to follow them. There won't be a need to rebel! Shape DIRTY, LAZY, KETO to work for you on *your own terms.* I grant you complete authority to claim recipes you enjoy and abandon those you don't like. Instead of following a prescribed meal plan, eat foods that make sense for your own body, not someone else's.

If you don't like a recipe, move on to the next one. If you hate a certain ingredient, substitute it for something you actually enjoy.

Make DIRTY, LAZY, KETO work for you. Flexibility is the key to success, my friend. Once you realize this, you are ready to start!

SHOPPING LISTS

I am providing you with my family's secret shopping list for inspiration. By no means are you required to run out and purchase everything I recommend. My shopping list is meant to give you some new ideas or inspiration to revisit old favorites. It took me *years* to identify DIRTY, LAZY, KETO foods at the grocery store, and I want to save you that time and effort.

You will notice a few things about my grocery list. First, I don't recommend a lot of *packaged foods*. I try to shop on the perimeter of the grocery store, where the "real food" is located. Fruits, vegetables, dairy, and meats tend to be stocked along the walls of any given grocery store. In general, the bulk of my diet consists of eating real foods that aren't heavily processed.

This isn't to say I don't enjoy a treat every once in a while. I love an Atkins bar or a bag of Quest Chips just as much as the next gal, but I have learned not to depend on these snacks for survival. These keto treats are often pricey and disappointing in taste, and worse, leave me still feeling hungry (and maybe constipated if I'm being 100 percent honest!).

> Eating DIRTY, LAZY, KETO is affordable. You don't need to buy anything fancy.

Second, you might observe my shopping list recommends full-fat items, especially in the dairy department. While this might seem counterintuitive to someone trying to lose weight, eating full-fat foods is a pivotal component of the DIRTY, LAZY, KETO way of eating. The explanation behind this metabolic miracle is discussed in detail throughout my first book, *DIRTY, LAZY, KETO: Get Started Losing Weight While Breaking the Rules*. Fat is satiating; it helps improve the taste of healthy foods. On DIRTY, LAZY, KETO, butter makes every vegetable taste like a rock star!

Last, you might be surprised about how many sugar-free foods are on my list. Did you even know some of these exist? Beginners sometimes assume they have to order "all things keto" online from expensive nutrition outlets in order to get started. This couldn't be further from the truth. You might be surprised that major discount retailers such as Walmart and Target, of all places, stock the majority of foods I recommend. While sugar-free foods might be hidden in the diabetic section by the pharmacy, they are still available on the shelf nonetheless. If you're like me, and super cost-conscious, you might discover even better prices by exploring the halls of discount retailers such as T.J. Maxx, Marshalls, Ross, dollar stores, and Big Lots, and of course by ordering online.

I often get emails from fans asking if a particular food is "keto" or not. I chuckle at this question! If the food is important to you, find a way to eat it.

> A unique benefit of DIRTY, LAZY, KETO is that it doesn't include self-deprivation. Count the carbs of your favorite foods in your planned net carb spend or find a satisfying keto substitute. *Empower yourself to make this work.*

Similarly, you might read over my grocery list and gasp about a recommendation. *This happens a lot from Strict Keto dropouts as they have been scorned.* "Onions! Garlic! But those have carbs!" they yell at the page. Yes, you are correct! This is *not* a zero-carb diet. I recommend you enjoy flavorful, high-fiber, yet healthy ingredients to make DIRTY, LAZY, KETO enjoyable and sustainable.

> No one has ever gotten fat from eating onions, my friend. Let's keep it real.

What about brands? Unless the recommended food item is unique, like Carbquik for example, I rarely recommend a specific brand. Personally, I buy whatever is on sale, and therefore I am not particularly brand loyal. Be sure to check the label of whatever foods you buy, however, as retailers and companies absolutely vary their ingredients, causing the carb count to potentially change. Because brands are inconsistent, always read the nutrition label on what you buy to prevent any surprises.

DIRTY, LAZY, KETO Grocery List

Note: Net carbs are provided per serving size and as a courtesy. Branded, packaged goods can vary with ingredients, so be sure to check the package's nutrition label to avoid any surprises.

DAIRY

Butter	0g net carbs
Cheese (all kinds)	1g net carbs
Cottage cheese (4% milk fat)	4g net carbs
Cream cheese (full-fat)	2g net carbs
Ghee	0g net carbs
Half and half (full fat)	1g net carbs
Heavy whipping cream (HWC)	1g net carbs
Ricotta cheese, whole milk (if needed for a planned recipe)	2g net carbs
Sour cream (full-fat)	1g net carbs
Unsweetened dairy alternative milk	1–6g net carbs
Whipped cream in the can (the real deal—for emergencies!)	1g net carbs
Yogurt (plain, full-fat, unsweetened—check label)	6–10g net carbs

PROTEIN

Bacon (avoid maple sugar flavor)	1g net carbs
Chicken (all parts, your preference)	0g net carbs
Deli meats (check labels as some brands add sugar)	1g net carbs
Duck	0g net carbs
Eggs	1g net carbs
Gyro meat (beef, lamb)	5g net carbs
Hot dogs (estimated, varies per brand)	2g net carbs
Lamb	0g net carbs
Lean meats (ground turkey, sausage, steak, and so on)	1g net carbs
Pepperoni	1g net carbs
Rotisserie chicken (avoid anything coated in barbecue sauce)	0g net carbs
Seafood (fish, shrimp, shellfish, lobster, but avoid fake crab)	1g net carbs
Soy chorizo	5–7g net carbs
Tofu (I prefer extra firm)	1–2g net carbs

PRODUCE

Artichokes	5g net carbs
Asparagus	2g net carbs
Avocados	2g net carbs
Bamboo shoots	5g net carbs
Beans (mung, green, wax, Italian)	2g net carbs
Bean sprouts	4g net carbs
Blueberries	18g net carbs
Broccoli	6g net carbs
Brussels sprouts	3g net carbs
Cabbage (green)	3g net carbs
Cabbage (bok choy)	1g net carbs
Cauliflower (riced, in bag)	2g net carbs
Cauliflower	3g net carbs
Celery	1g net carbs
Chayote	4g net carbs
Coleslaw	3g net carbs
Cucumbers	2g net carbs
Daikon radish	3g net carbs
Greens (collard)	3g net carbs
Greens (kale)	1g net carbs
Green beans	4g net carbs
Green onion	1g net carbs
Hearts of palm	3g net carbs
Herbs (fresh); except parsley which is 2g net carbs per 1 cup	0g net carbs
Jalapeños	1g net carbs
Jicama	5g net carbs
Leeks (cooked)	7g net carbs

PRODUCE	
Lemon	4g net carbs
Lettuce and salad mixes	1–2g net carbs
Lime	5g net carbs
Mushrooms	1g net carbs
Nuts (hazelnut, Brazil, pecan, macadamia, walnut, coconut)	4–7g net carbs
Pea pods (snow peas)	7g net carbs
Pepperoncini	0–1g net carbs
Radishes	2g net carbs
Raspberries	7g net carbs
Red onions	12g net carbs
Rhubarb	3g net carbs
Rutabaga (raw)	9g net carbs
Salad greens	0–1g net carbs
Seeds (chia, flax, pumpkin, sesame, sunflower)	5–11g net carbs
Shredded coleslaw/cabbage mix	3g net carbs
Snap peas	3g net carbs
Soybeans	5g net carbs
Spinach	1g net carbs
Sprouts (alfalfa)	0g net carbs
Star fruit	3g net carbs
Strawberries	8g net carbs
Swiss chard	2g net carbs
Tomatillos	1g net carbs
Tomato	5g net carbs
White onions	12g net carbs
Yellow onion	12g net carbs
Zucchini	1g net carbs

DRINKS

Coffee and tea	0g net carbs
Diet soda	0–2g net carbs
Electrolyte water (sugar-free)	0–1g net carbs
Flavored seltzer waters (sugar-free)	0g net carbs
Hard alcohol—unflavored (tequila, vodka, gin, whiskey, scotch, rum, brandy, cognac)	0g net carbs
Low-carb beers (Michelob Ultra, Corona Premier)	3–5g net carbs
Nonfat hot cocoa (strangely, this has fewer carbs than sugar-free hot cocoa)	4g net carbs
Sugar-free energy drinks	0–3g net carbs
Sugar-free water flavoring packets (or squirts)	0–1g net carbs

BAKING

Almond flour	3g net carbs
Chocolate bar (100% cocoa)	1g net carbs
Chocolate bar (92% cocoa)	6g net carbs
Chocolate bar (85% cocoa)	8g net carbs
Cocoa powder unsweetened	1g net carbs
Coconut flour	4g net carbs
Flaxseed meal	1g net carbs
Oil (coconut oil, olive oil, peanut oil, sesame oil)	0g net carbs
Protein powder (check carbs as brands vary)	2–5g net carbs
Pure vanilla extract	0g net carbs
Soy flour	5g net carbs
Sugar substitute (Splenda, Swerve, monk fruit, and so on)	0–1g net carbs
Sugar-free Jell-O gelatin powders	0g net carbs
Unsweetened shredded coconut	1g net carbs
Vital wheat gluten (used rarely in bread substitute recipes)	3g net carbs
Xanthan gum (used to thicken sauce, soup, or gravy)	0g net carbs

SAUCES AND SPICES

Everything but the Bagel spice (unnecessary, but delicious!)	0g net carbs
Au jus gravy mix powder	1g net carbs
Bouillon cubes	0–1g net carbs
Cinnamon (ground)	0g net carbs
Curry powder	0g net carbs
Flavored syrups (sugar-free) in coffee aisle	0–1g net carbs
Hot sauce (check label)	0g net carbs
Ketchup (no-sugar-added)	1g net carbs
Marinara sauce (no-sugar-added)	4g net carbs
Mayonnaise (full-fat)	0g net carbs
Mustard (yellow, spicy, and dry)	0g net carbs
Ranch powder mix	1g net carbs
Salad dressing (ranch, blue cheese; check label)	1–3g net carbs
Soy sauce	1g net carbs
Sriracha sauce	1g net carbs
Sugar-free pancake syrup	0g net carbs
Turmeric powder	0g net carbs
Vinegar (apple cider vinegar, plain white)	0g net carbs
Worcestershire sauce	1g net carbs

CANS AND JARS	
Alfredo sauce (fresh)	4g net carbs
Canned coconut milk (unsweetened, check label)	6–8g net carbs
Canned pumpkin	6–8g net carbs
Canned tuna	0g net carbs
Nut butter or no-sugar-added peanut butter	4–6g net carbs
Olives (green and black)	0g net carbs
Pesto (fresh)	2g net carbs
Pickles (not sweet/sour, unless you purchase "sugar-free")	2g net carbs
Sugar-free barbecue sauce	2g net carbs
Sugar-free jam	2g net carbs
MISCELLANEOUS	
Low-carb tortillas (occasional splurge)	4–6g net carbs
Pork rinds (I don't like these myself, but my husband loves them in recipes)	0g net carbs
Protein bars (occasionally, check label)	2–4g net carbs
Sugar-free candy (for emergencies!)	0–1g net carbs
Sugar-free gum	0g net carbs
Textured vegetable protein (TVP) (used rarely)	3–4g net carbs

I rarely purchase keto ingredients online as most are readily available in my local grocery stores. That being said, I have yet to find the following items at local stores.

ONLINE PURCHASES	
Black soybeans canned	1g net carbs
Carbquik baking mix	2g net carbs
MCT oil	0g net carbs

BROKE KETO

Organic vegetables, grass-fed beef, cage-free eggs, and line-caught fish… The source and style of food you buy is your business, my friend. I do not dare to judge your family's budget or belief system. Too often, we read diet books that insist ingredients must be of the "highest quality available" (often translating to outrageous prices). Strict standards about how food is sourced make me feel inadequate and even ashamed about what's inside my refrigerator. Even if I empathize with the cause, I often can't afford these foods obtained in these more respectable ways.

> I am not going to feel embarrassed about buying food from discount retailers like Walmart. I am proud I can feed my family!

Should I not save for Disney World this year and instead buy groceries only from a co-op? (I'm not even sure what that is.) My kids need braces and new shoes—should I substitute my family's financial priorities for grass-fed beef and free-range chicken for dinner? You bet I empathize with the plight of the farm animal, but not at the expense of paying rent.

> I may sound like the Jerry Springer of keto, but I want to be clear: Spending more money on groceries will not help you lose weight any faster.

To sum up, I want to assure you this is a judgment-free zone. Shop where you feel comfortable. Spend within your budget. No one here will question your belief system.

SUPPLIES AND A SASSY PANTS ATTITUDE

People often ask, "What do I need to get started?" All you *really* need is a positive attitude and a willingness to try (and fail) and try (and fail). Learning how to eat differently takes time. Remember, it took years upon years to gain your weight, I suspect, and it will also take some time to lose it. Be patient with yourself!

Don't beat yourself up over making a mistake. Failure is the most effective teacher.

> Beyond a willingness to try, you really need only the basics: a kitchen with a working fridge and a place to cook.

Having fancy culinary gadgets is unnecessary, but admittedly sometimes they make cooking more fun. I'm the first to admit that having a fancy new cooking tool might provide much-needed motivation. As a former teacher, I'm no stranger to positive reinforcement techniques. I'm definitely not above "bribing myself" with rewards. For example, after I log four hundred miles on my running shoes, I promise myself an upgraded pair of shoes! Bribes work in the kitchen too.

Sometimes gadgets that streamline healthy eating are worth the investment. For example, I love to eat hard-boiled eggs, but when I boil them on the stove, the stupid eggs either end up breaking or undercooked. Because of my "egg issues," investing in an Instant Pot® was worthwhile to me. I chose the one with a fancy yogurt-making feature in case I got the urge to take my cooking to the next level. (Note that I have yet to make homemade yogurt, *but someday people, I just might!*) I was also surprised that this handy device effortlessly steams vegetables and quickly cooks meat (even frozen meat!) at warp speed. I admit to initially being a little scared to use this spaceship-looking device. After watching a couple of *YouTube* videos, however, I quickly got the hang of it. The Instant Pot® is a game changer. Though costly, it has simplified my cooking and reduced the time I need to spend in the kitchen.

I thought my pressure cooker might replace my slow cooker as a personal favorite, but so far, that's not the case. With soups and stews, the slow cooker wins hands down. It's just so easy to throw in all of my ingredients and then *walk away*! I suspect my Instant Pot® offers a slow-cooking feature also, but that might still be too complicated for me. I have a long-standing love affair with my crusty, beloved slow cooker with an old-school plastic knob to turn toward low, high, or off. SIMPLE! I can handle that.

Except for these two cooking gadgets, the rest of my recommendations are pretty standard. To be thorough, however, I'll give you my list here:

+ **Ziploc bags.** Buy every size available of Ziploc bags and in quantities by the truckload. Ziploc bags are the best invention *ever*! Who still uses those fold-over plastic bags? My husband, that's who! He is the last person in America without a spill-proof lunch. In my opinion, Ziploc-branded bags are worth the extra expense.
+ **Tupperware.** Every year on Black Friday, I venture out during the wee hours to purchase a supersized gift pack of matching Tupperware. I get so much joy out of having the same size containers stack perfectly in my fridge. I must have some OCD issues, as I become absolutely disjointed when I come upon a drawer of ill-fitting, incompatible plastic containers. I give you permission to recycle your mismatched garbage and invest in a replacement set. Make your meal prep easy, safe, and attractive. I have even "upped my Tupperware game" by adding glass bowls with snap-on lids. Now I can safely microwave food without fears of BPA plastic melting all over my vegetables.
+ **Small cutting boards.** Who still uses a giant wooden block? When is the last time that thing was washed? I recommend that you purchase a set of small plastic cutting boards that can regularly become sanitized in the dishwasher. Making food prep simple and fast is the goal here, *not contracting salmonella.*
+ **Reusable water bottles.** Whether you are trendy like my teenager carrying an insulated Hydro Flask, or retro like me with a recycled glass bottle I can toss into the dishwasher, do yourself a favor and invest in a container that motivates you to drink lots of water. Water is truly the magic elixir to your weight loss.
+ **Colanders.** I am constantly washing fruits and vegetables, and often use both metal and plastic colanders of various sizes.
+ **Measuring cups and spoons.** I've been known to throw a meal together "Kentucky windage–style" (meaning no measuring), but not without consequence. Occasionally, my lack of specificity backfires and ruins my recipe! Be sure to have a set of

measuring cups and a set of measuring spoons on hand for accuracy or else your cheesecake might taste like gravel.

- **Nonstick cooking items.** A nonstick baking pan and/or round pizza pan, a nonstick baking mat, and parchment paper are essential tools in the DIRTY, LAZY, KETO kitchen. Can you think of anything worse than your homemade pizza becoming superglued to its pan?
- **Mini blender.** I just love my Bullet mini blender. I use it for smoothies, Bulletproof coffee, homemade pesto, and even cocktails. They are reasonably priced and sold with multiple blending cups that can be easily tossed into the dishwasher.
- **Immersion blender.** These are totally unnecessary, but so much fun. I use my immersion blender to whip Bulletproof coffee into a froth whenever I'm feeling the urge to be fancy. A few times a year, I'll use this to blend my soups (while they're still hot in the slow cooker). It's not a required cooking utensil by any means, but when you need it, you need it. Who wants to dump gallons of hot broccoli cheese soup into the blender for puréeing? *No one.* This "plug and play" tool does all the work and doesn't take up a lot of space. It's cheap too!

Conversely, I'd like to share a few kitchen items you *don't* need. If your kitchen counter space is anything like mine, there is absolutely no more room for another "life-changing appliance" to collect dust. With that in mind, go ahead and pass on the hot air popcorn popper and frozen yogurt machine. I'm sure those are fun devices to try (along with the bread maker of the 1980s), but all my useless kitchen appliances are collecting dust out in the garage.

TROUBLEMAKERS: FOODS TO AVOID

As you try and wrap your mind around what a DIRTY, LAZY, KETO recipe might look like, I want to give you a heads-up on ways I recommend "swapping out" your starches. I know when I first started DIRTY, LAZY, KETO, I was desperate to find *the perfect alternative* to bread. Sadly (I have to give it to you straight right now), a perfect substitute does not exist! You can try all the different cloud bread and chaffle recipes in the world, but they will *never exactly* mimic the taste of fresh bread. Go ahead and get angry. Be sad even. You may even need to take a break from reading and properly mourn the loss of your favorite sandwich staple.

It wasn't until I lowered my bread expectations and said goodbye to the starch category that I became truly happy. You can't live in the past, my friend. "Let it go!"

Here is a list of high-starch foods to avoid. All of these net carb counts are "per serving" and are estimates/generalizations using all the information available to the authors at the time.

HIGH-STARCH FOODS	
Bagels	55g net carbs
Bananas	27g net carbs
Beer	12g net carbs
Biscuits	16g net carbs
Black beans	40g net carbs per cup
Brown rice	46g net carbs
Corn	16g net carbs
Commercial bread	13–20g net carbs
Cookies	18g net carbs
Corn flakes cereal	24g net carbs per cup
Doughnuts	22g net carbs
Flour tortillas	24g net carbs
Grits	38g net carbs
Hash browns	26g net carbs
Ice cream	16g net carbs

HIGH-STARCH FOODS	
Low-fat milk	12g net carbs
Muffins (blueberry)	48g net carbs
Oatmeal	27g net carbs per cup
Orange juice	26g net carbs
Pancakes	40g net carbs
Pasta	32g net carbs
Peas	21g net carbs
Potato chips	15g net carbs
Potatoes	37g net carbs
Pretzels	23g net carbs
Quinoa	39g net carbs
Refried beans	68g net carbs per cup
Saltine crackers (12)	26g net carbs
Sweet potato	26g net carbs
Sweetened yogurt	32g net carbs
White flour	95g net carbs per cup
White rice	44g net carbs

Training Wheels: Foods to Help with Transition

These foods can help you as you transition to a reduced-carb diet, but keep in mind that they are specialty items and are often pricey.

TRANSITION FOODS	
Hearts of palm pasta (never tried due to *outrageous* price)	4g net carbs
Low-carb tortillas (rubbery, but I still like them!)	4–6g net carbs
Shirataki noodles (so fishy!)	1g net carbs
ThinSlim bread (Aldi and other brands, pricey and hard to find)	0g net carbs

THE BIG LEAGUES: YOUR KETO STAPLES

These foods are inexpensive and readily available. These foods are low in carbs and common enough that you should always have most of these on hand to serve as a side dish or a quick snack to satisfy your hunger right away and prevent a potentially destructive carb relapse. These net carb amounts are "per serving."

VEGETABLE STAPLES	
Boiled radishes (seriously! we will get to this later)	2g net carbs
Cauliflower rice	1g net carbs
Celery stalks	1g net carbs
Green beans	4g net carbs
Grilled eggplant	3g net carbs
Jicama fries	3g net carbs
Lettuce wraps	0g net carbs
Mixed greens/lettuce	1g net carbs
Portabella mushrooms	2g net carbs
Steamed cauliflower	1g net carbs
"Zoodles" or sliced zucchini	1g net carbs

Sugar and Flour Substitutes

SUGAR SUBSTITUTES		
Acesulfame-K (Ace-K)	Sweet One	1g net carbs per packet 1g net carbs per gram
Aspartame	Equal NutraSweet	0g net carbs per teaspoon 1g net carbs per packet
Erythritol blended with oligosaccharides	Swerve	0g net carbs per teaspoon 0g net carbs per packet 0g net carbs per 1 gram
Monk fruit (luo han guo)	Monk Fruit In The Raw Nature's Nectresse PureFruit Swanson PureLo	0g net carbs per packet 0g net carbs per packet 0g net carbs per gram
Organic raw coconut sugar		3g net carbs per teaspoon 1g net carbs per packet 1g net carbs per gram
Saccharin	Necta Sweet Sweet'N Low Sugar Twin	1g net carbs per packet 1g net carbs per gram 1g net carbs per gram
Steviol glycosides	SweetLeaf Stevia Pure Via Stevia In the Raw Truvia	1g net carbs per packet 1g net carbs per gram
Sucralose	Splenda	1g net carbs per packet 1g net carbs per gram
SUGAR (FOR REFERENCE)		
Honey		6g net carbs per teaspoon 1g net carbs per gram
White table sugar		4g net carbs per teaspoon 3g net carbs per packet 1g net carbs per gram

FLOUR SUBSTITUTES

Almond flour, fine	2g net carbs per ½ cup
Carbquik Baking Mix	2g net carbs per ⅓ cup
Coconut flour	3–12g net carbs per ½ cup, depending on brand
Flaxseed meal	0–2g net carbs per tablespoon, depending on brand
Parmesan cheese	1g net carbs per tablespoon
Pork rinds	0g net carbs per 1 cup
Psyllium husk powder	0–1g net carbs per tablespoon, depending on brand
Soy flour	6–9g net carbs per ½ cup, depending on brand
Vital wheat gluten	3g net carbs per ¼ cup

WHITE FLOUR (FOR REFERENCE)

All-purpose enriched white flour	46g net carbs per ½ cup

THE DIRTY, LAZY, KETO RECIPES

Look What's Cookin'

CHAPTER 3

BREAKFAST

Let the games begin! I don't know about you, but I could eat breakfast foods ALL DAY LONG. There is a *"carboliciousness"* associated with morning foods that has warmed my heart for decades. I adore sweet cereals, warm breads, salty fats, and of course, *syrup*! I'm so happy DIRTY, LAZY, KETO meets my romantic breakfast desires, or I might have gone back to the dark side.

There is something so satisfying about starting the day off with something sweet. When I was breastfeeding my newborn daughter, I would spend all morning in a fluffy yellow chair sipping a quart of cranberry juice while gnawing on sweet rolls. Oh, how I loved those Swedish-style cinnamon snails! Would it surprise you to hear that I gained more weight AFTER my baby was born than during my pregnancy? Clearly, I took the notion that "breastfeeding burns a lot of calories" to the next level. *Was I feeding an army of newborns or just one?*

Even though my baby is now a teenager, my morning sweet tooth persists. As I've mentioned before, I recommend working *with* your habits, not against them. When you catch yourself saying, "Oh, but I should…" a little bell needs to go off. There is nothing wrong with your current habits, only the doughnuts you might be consuming to nurture them. I want you to fully enjoy your sweet-and-salty breakfast, but do it DIRTY, LAZY, KETO style!

FLAPPA JACKS $ ⚝ ✕ 🌿

NET CARBS

3G

SERVES 6

PER SERVING:

CALORIES	273
FAT	23G
PROTEIN	10G
SODIUM	202MG
FIBER	4G
CARBOHYDRATES	7G
SUGAR	2G

TIME

PREP TIME:	10 MIN
COOK TIME:	14 MIN

TIPS & OPTIONS ≫

I have been known to add a little "flair" like sugar-free chocolate chips or even finely crushed peppermint candy to the batter of my Flappa Jacks.

Food coloring can be added during the holidays (or anytime). You can even get creative with sizes and shapes.

Sometimes while making Flappa Jacks for the entire family, I get tired of making the typical-sized pancakes (2"–4") and just want to get it over with! I've been known to make supersized pancakes just to finish off the batter.

For years, my husband and I enjoyed "All You Can Eat Pancake Day" at IHOP. We were such frequent visitors that the waitress soon remembered every detail of our orders. I don't know if I should be flattered or offended by that kind of attention! Clearly, I liked me some pancakes! I still have trouble controlling myself around these keto Flappa Jacks, as I will unnecessarily overeat any kind of pancake until my tummy pokes out and I can barely breathe. In case you have more self-control than I do, here is my favorite recipe for Flappa Jacks. Enjoy these delicious gems with butter and sugar-free syrup.

1 cup blanched almond flour

¼ cup coconut flour

5 large eggs, whisked

3 (1-gram) packets 0g net carb sweetener

1 teaspoon baking powder

⅓ cup unsweetened almond milk

¼ cup vegetable oil

1½ teaspoons pure vanilla extract

⅛ teaspoon salt

1. In a large mixing bowl, mix all ingredients together until smooth.

2. In a large nonstick skillet over medium heat, pour desired-sized pancakes and cook 3–5 minutes until bubbles form.

3. Flip pancakes and cook another 2 minutes until brown. Repeat as needed to use all batter. Serve.

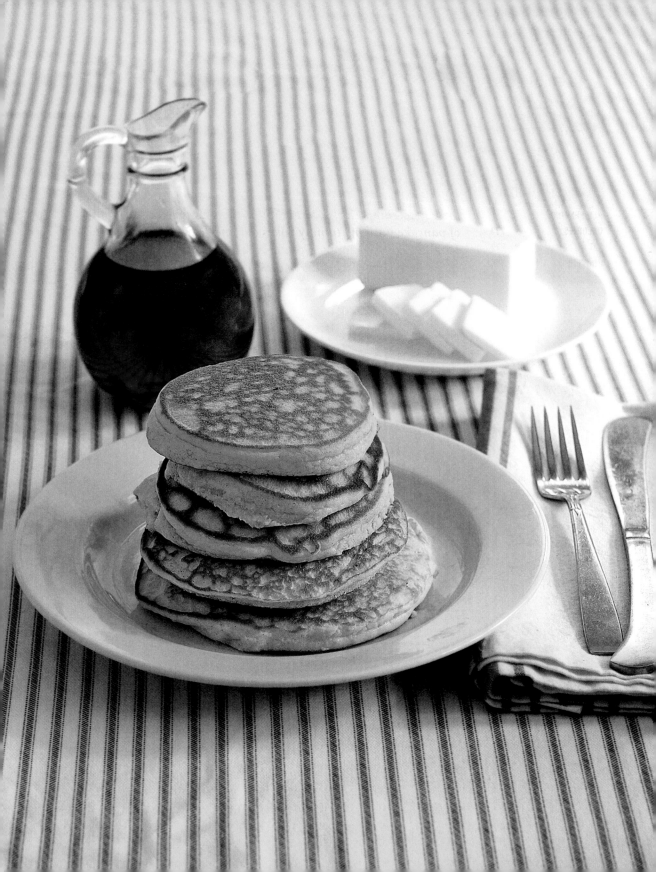

BOOGA CHIA CEREAL $

NET CARBS

2G

SERVES 1

PER SERVING:

CALORIES	132
FAT	9G
PROTEIN	4G
SODIUM	93MG
FIBER	9G
CARBOHYDRATES	11G
SUGAR	0G

TIME

PREP TIME: 2 MIN +
REFRIGERATION OVERNIGHT
COOK TIME: 0 MIN

TIPS & OPTIONS ⟫

I recommend making multiple servings at once. I make five single-serving batches in small reusable containers and stack them in the refrigerator to last the entire week.

Chia cereal can be enjoyed cold or warmed in the microwave.

Top with a handful of walnuts, pecans, or even sugar-free chocolate chips for added variety. Sprinkle a dash of unsweetened shredded coconut or cinnamon on top for taste and color.

Beware: Chia seeds can be constipating!

Warm your chia cereal in the microwave for 1 minute, and *DAMN* if it won't remind you of Cream of Wheat!

I spent years forsaking a morning bowl of cereal while trying to lose weight. Once I discovered chia cereal, however, my DIRTY, LAZY, KETO life was forever changed for the better. Why did I wait so long to try chia seeds? Well, first of all, I thought the consistency was "creepy." Like a runny jam, chia seeds swell when mixed with liquid. They start off as inedible, tiny hard balls, but blossom into a tapioca-like consistency when liquid is added. After I finally took the plunge to try this "boogery" concoction, I was pleasantly surprised. **Chia seeds are actually delicious!**

2 tablespoons chia seeds

2 (1-gram) packets 0g net carb sweetener

½ cup unsweetened almond milk

⅛ teaspoon pure vanilla extract

1   Add all ingredients to a small container or bowl. Stir until blended.

2   Let soak overnight in refrigerator for best results as chia seeds soften as they absorb liquid and swell.

3   Serve the next morning.

SAWDUST OATMEAL $ ★ 🌱

Grain-free "noatmeal" is a fast way to get your morning started on the right note. If you love grits, Sawdust Oatmeal will quickly become your new DIRTY, LAZY, KETO grits replacement. The flaxseed meal ingredient provides that gritty texture. Similar to traditional grits, this cereal has oodles of fiber that will do wonders for your constitution.

⅓ cup boiling water

2 tablespoons chia seeds

2 tablespoons flaxseed meal

2 tablespoons heavy whipping cream

1 (1-gram) packet 0g net carb sweetener

1 Add all ingredients to a small glass or porcelain bowl. Stir to mix. Be careful as water is very hot.

2 Stir every couple of minutes as it cools to ensure even cooling. The chia seeds soften and expand as they absorb liquid.

3 When it's cool, it's ready to eat.

NET CARBS
4G

SERVES 1	
PER SERVING:	
CALORIES	289
FAT	22G
PROTEIN	8G
SODIUM	14MG
FIBER	11G
CARBOHYDRATES	15G
SUGAR	1G

TIME	
PREP TIME:	5 MIN
COOK TIME:	0 MIN

TIPS & OPTIONS

Top with a handful of berries, walnuts, pecans, or even sugar-free chocolate chips for added variety.

Nut butter is another great addition to stir in.

Chia seeds can be constipating!

Let the chia seeds sit for at least an hour to fully absorb the water and soften.

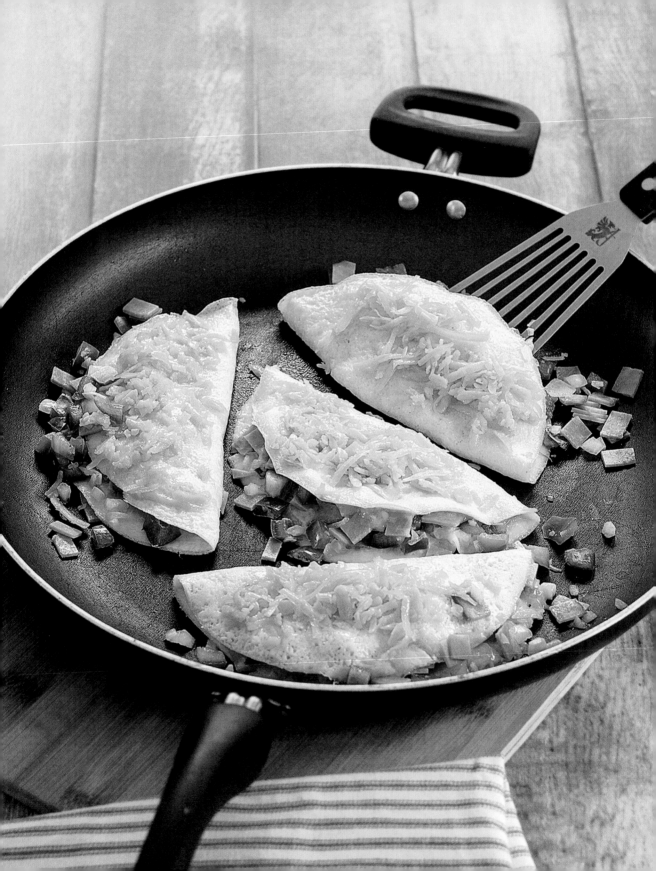

WEEKEND WESTERN OMELET $ 🍴

Whether eggs are prepared in the microwave or in a cast iron skillet, I love to eat them for their simplicity, nutritious boost, and flexibility to incorporate vegetables. I tend to prepare my eggs on the stovetop only on the weekends (as this requires additional time and cleanup on my part). During the weekdays, I take a shortcut by eating microwaved scrambled eggs on a paper plate while driving to work—gasp!

8 large eggs

10 ounces smoked ham, finely chopped

4 tablespoons heavy whipping cream

1 small yellow onion, peeled and chopped

1 small green bell pepper, seeded and chopped

8 tablespoons unsalted butter, divided

1 cup shredded Cheddar cheese, divided

1 In a large bowl, whisk eggs and mix in the ham and cream.

2 In a medium microwave-safe bowl, microwave the onion and pepper for 3 minutes.

3 In a medium skillet over medium-low heat, melt 2 tablespoons butter and quickly pour one-quarter of the egg mixture into skillet before it separates.

4 After 4–5 minutes, when entire bottom of egg mixture has cooked, add one-quarter of onion and pepper to center of omelet.

5 Use spatula to fold egg mixture in half onto itself. Let omelet finish cooking another 3–4 minutes.

6 Slide the fully cooked omelet onto a warmed plate. Top with one-quarter of shredded cheese.

7 Repeat process three more times for the remaining three omelets.

NET CARBS

3G

SERVES 4

PER SERVING:

CALORIES	593
FAT	46G
PROTEIN	32G
SODIUM	1,193MG
FIBER	1G
CARBOHYDRATES	4G
SUGAR	2G

TIME

PREP TIME:	10 MIN
COOK TIME:	39 MIN

》 TIPS & OPTIONS

Add additional vegetables to your diet by experimenting with adding an assortment of low-carb vegetables.

The green bell pepper has the least amount of carbs of all the different colored bell peppers.

With a sprinkle of last night's leftover vegetables inside your omelet, you won't even realize your breakfast just got "healthier."

The varieties of omelets are endless; be brave!

CHRISTMAS SOUFFLÉ $ ◉ ✕

NET CARBS

3G

SERVES 6

PER SERVING:

CALORIES	287
FAT	21G
PROTEIN	16G
SODIUM	475MG
FIBER	1G
CARBOHYDRATES	4G
SUGAR	2G

TIME

PREP TIME:	10 MIN
COOK TIME:	35 MIN

TIPS & OPTIONS ⟫

Make your soufflé vegetarian-"ish" by omitting meat and adding vegetables only.

Want a kick in the pants? Spicy food lovers can opt to add chopped jalapeño to their soufflé for added punch.

On Christmas Eve I prepare this colorful egg dish, tucking it safely into the fridge for Santa's arrival. Before my family starts opening up presents on Christmas morning, I pop the soufflé into the oven. Breakfast is soon ready without me having to lift a finger! I slice the soufflé into squares and serve to my family while we sit around the Christmas tree. While technically the soufflé may not rise to the level of Julia Child's expectations, for me, the ability to open gifts with my children instead of slaving away in the kitchen is worth any culinary sacrifice.

½ tablespoon olive oil

1 medium onion, peeled and finely chopped

1½ teaspoons minced garlic

6 large eggs, whisked

6 ounces cured ham, finely cubed

1 cup shredded Cheddar cheese

½ cup heavy whipping cream

½ cup finely chopped tomato

½ cup finely chopped green onion

1   Preheat oven to 400°F. Grease a 9" × 9" baking dish.

2   In a medium nonstick pan over medium heat, add oil, onion, and garlic. Cook 3–5 minutes while stirring until brown and soft. Remove from heat.

3   In a large mixing bowl, mix all ingredients. Pour into baking dish.

4   Bake 25–30 minutes until cooked all the way through.

5   Serve Christmas Soufflé while warm.

COUNTERFEIT BAGELS

I tried to make keto bagels several times without success. After the first round, my bagels looked like flat egg noodles! Even with the addition of baking powder to get a rise from my recipe, this self-proclaimed bagel addict still felt underwhelmed. Surprisingly, my family excitedly swarmed around these Counterfeit Bagels as they exited the oven. Apparently, the waft of warm bread doesn't escape my kitchen very often (or never, these days!). I figured if my children could be fooled into thinking these were real bagels, I could convince myself too. With a little cream cheese and a sprinkle of Everything but the Bagel seasoning, my senses were admittedly fooled!

1½ cups blanched almond flour

1 tablespoon baking powder

2½ cups shredded whole milk mozzarella cheese

2 ounces full-fat cream cheese, softened

2 large eggs, whisked

2 tablespoons Everything but the Bagel seasoning

1 tablespoon unsalted butter, melted

1 Preheat oven to 400°F. Line a baking sheet with parchment paper.

2 In a small bowl, mix almond flour and baking powder.

3 In a medium microwave-safe bowl, mix mozzarella cheese, cream cheese, and whisked eggs.

4 Microwave cheese mixture 1 minute. Stir and microwave again 30 seconds. Let mixture cool until okay to handle.

5 Combine dry ingredients into cheese mixture. Work quickly, stirring with a sturdy spatula or bamboo spoon to create dough. Shape dough into approximately ¾"-thick snakes, and then form into ten bagels.

6 Place bagels on prepared baking sheet and sprinkle tops with seasoning. Bake 15 minutes until browning on top.

7 Remove bagels from oven, brush with melted butter, and serve.

NET CARBS
3G

SERVES 10	
PER SERVING:	
CALORIES	236
FAT	18G
PROTEIN	11G
SODIUM	548MG
FIBER	2G
CARBOHYDRATES	5G
SUGAR	1G

TIME	
PREP TIME:	15 MIN
COOK TIME:	17 MIN

TIPS & OPTIONS

Top with cream cheese and sugar-free preserves. You're welcome!

Express yourself and add to the dough whatever suits your fancy; chopped nuts, diced jalapeño, or even sugar-free chocolate chips.

STARBUCKS EGG BITES $ ✕

I love egg bites because I can make them in large batches and easily freeze individual portions in Ziploc bags. In the morning, I pop a couple of egg bites in the microwave and VOILÀ! A fancy breakfast is served. I urge you to double or even triple this recipe as your family members will likely gobble them up (when you are not looking) and leave you with no leftovers. This recipe mimics the egg bites sold at Starbucks (but without all the added unnecessary potato starch).

5 large eggs, whisked

1 cup shredded Swiss cheese

1 cup full-fat cottage cheese

⅛ teaspoon salt

⅛ teaspoon black pepper

2 strips no-sugar-added bacon, cooked and crumbled

1 Preheat oven to 350°F.

2 In a large bowl, whisk together eggs, Swiss cheese, cottage cheese, salt, and pepper.

3 Pour six equal amounts of mixture into well-greased muffin tins (or use cupcake liners).

4 Top with bacon bits.

5 Bake 30 minutes until eggs are completely cooked.

6 Remove Starbucks Egg Bites from oven and serve warm.

NET CARBS

3G

SERVES 6

PER SERVING:

CALORIES	182
FAT	11G
PROTEIN	16G
SODIUM	321MG
FIBER	0G
CARBOHYDRATES	3G
SUGAR	1G

TIME

PREP TIME:	5 MIN
COOK TIME:	30 MIN

TIPS & OPTIONS ≫

Have fun trying out different varieties of egg bites. Whether it's ham and cheese, garden vegetable or broccoli and Cheddar, the combinations are endless.

Making egg bites at home, as opposed to purchasing in the drive-thru, keeps you in control of the ingredients. Your efforts will be rewarded as the homemade variety omits high-carb "fillers" that are commonplace in commercial production.

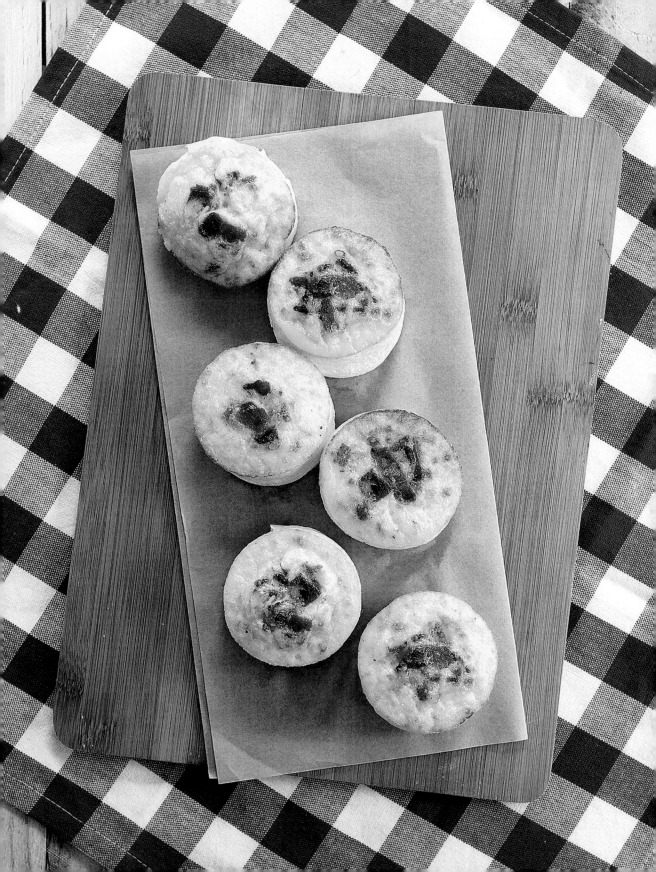

DLK BULLETPROOF COFFEE $

NET CARBS
0G

SERVES 1

PER SERVING:

CALORIES	132
FAT	14G
PROTEIN	0G
SODIUM	4MG
FIBER	0G
CARBOHYDRATES	0G
SUGAR	0G

TIME

PREP TIME:	2 MIN
COOK TIME:	0 MIN

TIPS & OPTIONS

Substitute MCT oil for a tablespoon of fat of your choosing: butter, coconut oil, half and half, or heavy whipping cream.

If you choose MCT oil as your added fat, use sparingly. MCT oil has a known laxative effect. *Less is more.*

Prefer your coffee sweet? Add a 0g net carb sweetener of your choice.

One warning: My friend Carol learned this one the hard way—her Styrofoam cup of coffee with MCT oil literally *exploded* in her hand! Apparently the MCT oil reacts with the Styrofoam, thus weakening and dissolving it.

The requirement to drink Bulletproof coffee is probably the biggest myth among keto followers. Repeat after me—this is not required! Some folks find that adding fats to their morning cup of joe helps to curb hunger (and therefore prolong the fast from the night before). Bulletproof coffee is simply a cup of coffee with a fat added, usually butter, MCT oil, or coconut oil. There is no right or wrong way to make DLK Bulletproof Coffee. Make and enjoy a blend that works best for your personal taste.

1 tablespoon MCT oil

8 ounces hot brewed coffee

1   Add MCT oil to coffee and blend using a hand immersion blender until froth whips up. This will help prevent the dreaded MCT oil *"lip gloss."*

2   Serve.

GREEN MONSTER SMOOTHIE $ ✕ 🌿

Smoothies are a refreshing way to "eat" your fruits and vegetables, especially if you struggle with their taste. Somehow, the blend of ice, sugar-free sweetener, and a creamy elixir makes just about any vegetable palatable. My kids, who scoff at eating steamed spinach, slurp down the Green Monster Smoothie without a second thought.

- 1 cup ice
- 1 cup chopped fresh spinach
- ½ cup fresh raspberries
- 2 (1-gram) packets 0g net carb sweetener
- 1 cup unsweetened almond milk (or dairy alternative milk of your choice)

Pulse all ingredients in a food processor or blender 30–60 seconds until ice is blended.

NET CARBS

4G

SERVES 1

PER SERVING:

CALORIES	67
FAT	3G
PROTEIN	3G
SODIUM	203MG
FIBER	6G
CARBOHYDRATES	10G
SUGAR	3G

TIME

PREP TIME:	3 MIN
COOK TIME:	0 MIN

TIPS & OPTIONS

Fresh or frozen spinach can be used. It's going to be blended anyhow! Fresh spinach just tastes better.

Add additional low-carb veggies, low-carb yogurt, and/or protein powder.

Depending on your personal taste, use more or less of the 0g net carb sweetener.

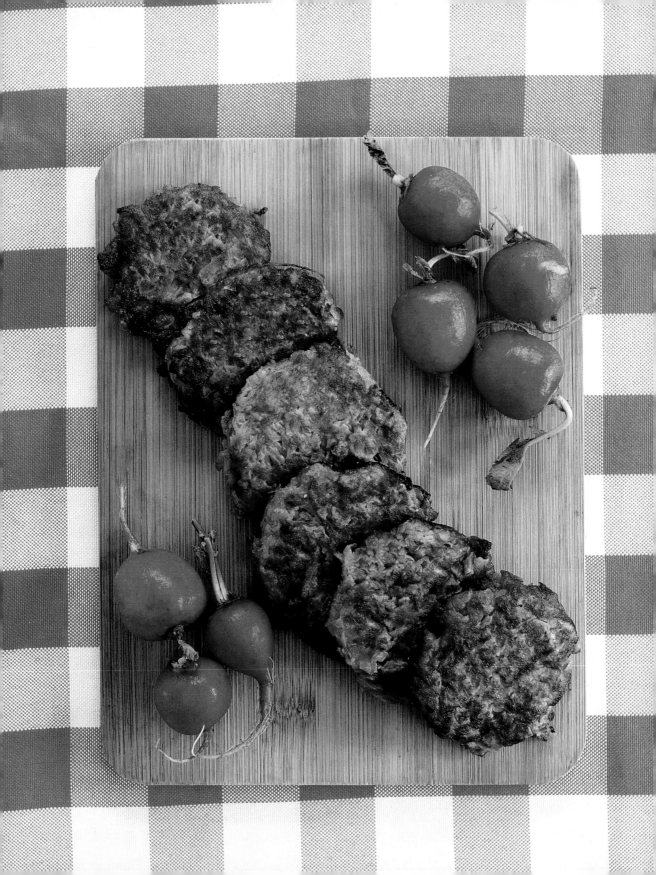

RADISH HASH BROWNS $

*While these may not taste like McDonald's hash browns, you still won't be disappointed. I continue to be **mystified** by how a bitter and crunchy radish can transform itself into a savory morning treat. The secret with radishes is to cook them well-done and add a lot of salt. WHO KNEW?*

2 pounds radishes, trimmed

4 tablespoons olive oil

1 large egg, whisked

⅛ teaspoon salt

⅛ teaspoon black pepper

1. Shred radishes using a food processor or hand grater and squeeze out extra moisture using cheesecloth or clean dish towel.

2. In a medium skillet over medium heat, heat oil. Add radishes and stir often. Sauté 20–30 minutes until golden. Remove from heat and place into a medium bowl.

3. Stir whisked egg into bowl with salt and pepper.

4. Form ten small pancakes. Add back to hot skillet. Heat 3–5 minutes on each side until solid and brown.

5. Serve warm.

NET CARBS
1G

SERVES 10

PER SERVING:

CALORIES	63
FAT	6G
PROTEIN	1G
SODIUM	58MG
FIBER	1G
CARBOHYDRATES	2G
SUGAR	1G

TIME

PREP TIME:	10 MIN
COOK TIME:	40 MIN

TIPS & OPTIONS

Radish Hash Browns pair perfectly with a Weekend Western Omelet (see recipe in this chapter).

I find that a sprinkle of shredded cheese or a dollop of sour cream makes the Radish Hash Browns quite tasty.

CHAPTER 4

SOUPS AND SALADS

"Lettuce" eat a lot! Salads have gotten a bad rap in the diet world. Most of us were brought up to believe that proper ladies nibbled on limp lettuce leaves to maintain girlish figures. As a result, we were programmed to think *salads equal deprivation and weight loss.* Well no longer, my friends! Let's talk about some hearty salads that include plenty of nutritious fiber but with all the healthy fats and proteins you need to be satisfied.

Something I love about salads and soups is the *volume.* There is nothing that gives me more happiness than filling a giant mixing bowl full of salad or soup that I can eat while binge-watching *Netflix.* Many an armchair psychologist is now throwing their hands in the air in exasperation. "THAT'S her problem! Mindless eating in front of the television…"

Yes, there might be some truth in that. But I decided long ago in my weight loss journey that I would work with myself, and not against. I don't have the time, desire, or resources to meet with a counselor to "fix" my problems. So, I have decided to just go with the flow. Eating relaxes me. Instead of unwinding with a bowl of Cheez-Its like I used to, however, I'm now digging into one of my patented DIRTY, LAZY, KETO favorite soup or salad recipes.

NO-GUILT VEGETABLE SOUP

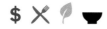

NET CARBS
6G

SERVES 12

PER SERVING:

CALORIES	153
FAT	5G
PROTEIN	16G
SODIUM	348MG
FIBER	4G
CARBOHYDRATES	10G
SUGAR	5G

TIME

PREP TIME:	20 MIN
COOK TIME:	35 MIN

TIPS & OPTIONS

Use any vegetable combination that suits you.

Make your soup even heartier by adding leftover cooked meat from last night's dinner.

Prefer a cream-based soup? Add more cream cheese or a tablespoon of half and half for creaminess.

To thicken your soup, add 1 teaspoon powdered xanthan gum, which acts as a strong, low-carb thickener. First, mix the xanthan in a separate bowl with a dribble of water until a gel is formed. Add to soup sparingly as *less is more.*

Need flexibility for non-keto family members? Separate part of the soup into a second pot and add pasta or rice.

*No-Guilt Vegetable Soup, aka "whatever you have on hand" vegetable soup, assuages your guilt over rotting produce. I buy a ton of vegetables every week. Since I shop at the dollar store (where vegetables cost, you guessed it, **a dollar!**), I sometimes go overboard. I tend to overbuy vegetables, with the hope that the bounty of healthy options will lead me down a better path. When vegetables start approaching expiration, I resuscitate their value by throwing them into the kitchen sink for a baptismal bath to bring them back to life. I feel too guilty throwing away vegetables!*

2 tablespoons vegetable oil

1 cup diced celery

1 small carrot, peeled and diced

1 medium head cauliflower, chopped into bite-sized florets

1 small eggplant, diced

2 cups finely cut broccoli florets

2 (64-ounce) cans chicken bone broth

1 cup cut green beans (cut into 1" sections)

2 medium zucchini, diced

1½ teaspoons dried basil

¼ teaspoon dried thyme leaves

1 teaspoon black pepper

¼ teaspoon dried sage

¼ teaspoon garlic salt

4 ounces full-fat cream cheese

1 In a large soup pot over medium heat, add oil and then sauté celery, carrot, cauliflower, eggplant, and broccoli until lightly softened (about 3–5 minutes), stirring regularly.

2 Add bone broth and remaining vegetables and spices.

3 Cover pot and bring to boil. Reduce heat and simmer 30 minutes until vegetables reach desired level of softness. Stir every 5 minutes.

4 Stir in cream cheese until fully blended.

5 Let cool 10 minutes and then serve.

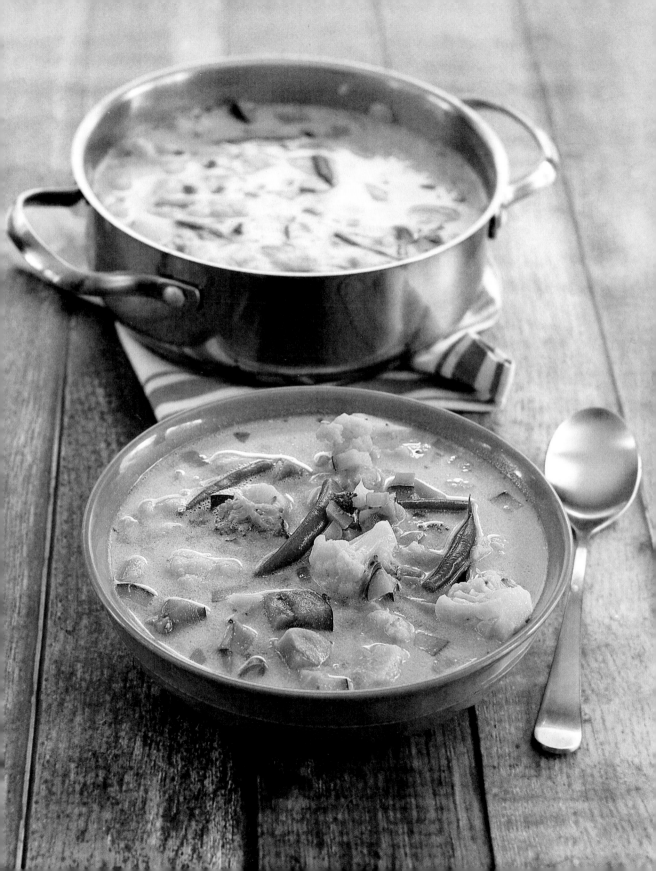

"DOLLA STORE" PUMPKIN SOUP $

NET CARBS

8G

SERVES 8

PER SERVING:

CALORIES	237
FAT	15G
PROTEIN	17G
SODIUM	818MG
FIBER	5G
CARBOHYDRATES	13G
SUGAR	3G

TIME

PREP TIME:	15 MIN
COOK TIME:	25 MIN

TIPS & OPTIONS »

Top with coconut yogurt or sour cream and pumpkin seeds if desired.

If substituting meat chorizo for the soy chorizo, brown the meat chorizo for 10–15 minutes and drain fat before adding to the pot.

For increased bulk, double the amount of vegetables by adding chopped zucchini.

To reduce carb amount, decrease the recipe's amount of pumpkin and increase quantity of cruciferous vegetables.

"Dolla Store" Pumpkin Soup is often served at my house on a lazy Sunday when the fridge is almost empty and payday is in the distant future. Many of these ingredients are found at our local dollar store, so this recipe ends up being very affordable as an added bonus! Canned pumpkin and tubes of soy chorizo for a dollar each? How fun is that? Cheap and delicious. I make this in my slow cooker and freeze leftovers for another day when I don't feel like cooking.

2 (9-ounce) packages soy chorizo

6 cups chicken bone broth

½ (15-ounce) can pure pumpkin

2 cups cooked riced cauliflower

1 cup unsweetened coconut milk

1 teaspoon garlic powder

1 teaspoon ground cinnamon

1 teaspoon ground ginger

1 teaspoon ground nutmeg

1 teaspoon paprika

⅛ teaspoon salt

⅛ teaspoon black pepper

1 Place a medium soup pot over medium heat and add all ingredients. Bring to boil while stirring regularly (5–10 minutes).

2 Reduce heat. Let simmer 15 minutes, stirring regularly until desired consistency achieved.

3 Remove from heat, let cool 5 minutes, and serve.

SLOW COOKER TACO BELL SOUP $ ✕ ⬛

If I didn't have a slow cooker, my family just might starve for half of the year. I have other things to do besides stand over a hot stove! In fact, I prefer having my slow cooker do all of the work while I catch up on Netflix. Slow Cooker Taco Bell Soup is one of my favorites due to its simplicity and speed (I need to get back to my show already). It has just the right amount of flavor to entice the entire family without being too spicy.

2 pounds lean ground beef

1 medium onion, peeled and chopped

2 cloves garlic, peeled and minced

6 cups beef broth

2 cups water

8 ounces full-fat cream cheese, cubed

½ cup finely chopped cilantro

2 (4-ounce) cans diced green chilies, drained

2 tablespoons taco seasoning

1 In a medium skillet over medium heat, brown ground beef 10–15 minutes while stirring. Drain fat. Add onion and garlic. Sauté 5 minutes.

2 Add meat mixture to slow cooker along with rest of ingredients.

3 Cover with lid and cook 2 hours on high or 4 hours on low.

4 Let cool 10 minutes and then serve.

NET CARBS
4G

SERVES 8

PER SERVING:

CALORIES	307
FAT	16G
PROTEIN	26G
SODIUM	1,089MG
FIBER	2G
CARBOHYDRATES	6G
SUGAR	3G

TIME

PREP TIME:	20 MIN
COOK TIME:	
HIGH TEMP....	2 HR 20 MIN
LOW TEMP	4 HR 20 MIN

《 TIPS & OPTIONS

Serve with your choice of toppings like olives, jalapeños, or a dollop of full-fat sour cream.

You can substitute any ground meat of your choice.

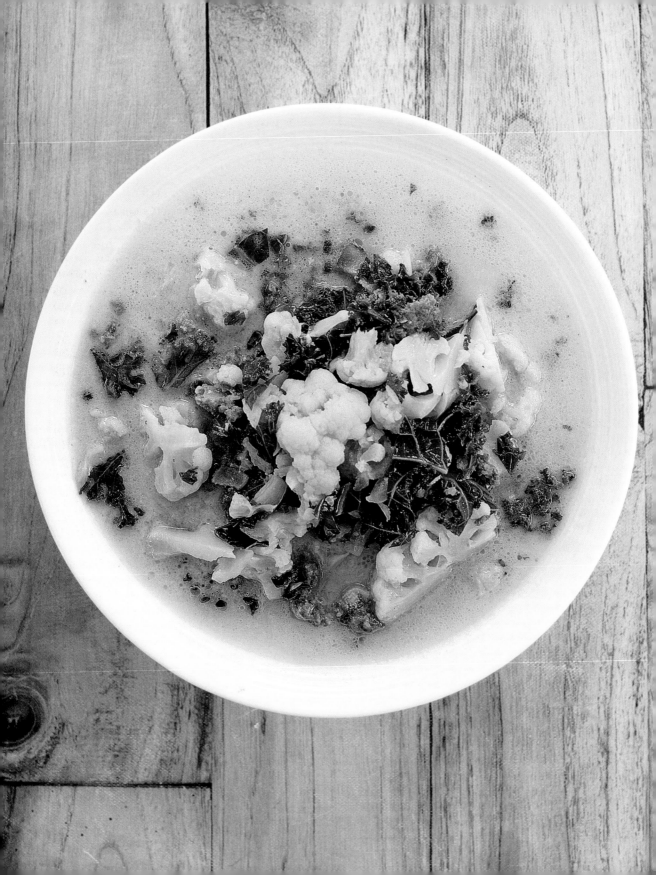

OG ZUPPA TOSCANA SOUP $

If you serve OG Zuppa Toscana Soup with the Olive Garden Salad (see recipe in this chapter) and OG Breadsticks recipe (Chapter 6), you won't ever have to leave the house again to get an Italian meal! This low-carb soup dish looks and tastes exactly like what you will find at the restaurant, leaving the potatoes (and high carbs!) behind.

1 pound loose Italian sausage

1 tablespoon unsalted butter

1½ cups chopped onion

3 cloves garlic, peeled and minced

8 cups water

2 (1 teaspoon) chicken bouillon cubes

½ pound no-sugar-added bacon, cooked and crumbled

4 cups chopped cauliflower, chopped into bite-sized chunks

4 cups chopped kale

1½ cups heavy whipping cream

1 In a medium-sized skillet over medium heat, cook sausage 10–15 minutes while stirring until brown. Drain fat.

2 In a large soup pot over medium heat, melt butter and then add onion. Sauté 3–5 minutes until soft and clear. Add garlic and cook 1 more minute. Add water and bouillon cubes.

3 Add crumbled bacon, cauliflower, and cooked sausage to pot.

4 When water reaches boil, reduce heat to low, cover pot, and simmer 15–20 minutes, stirring regularly until cauliflower reaches desired softness.

5 Add kale and cream. Cook, stirring regularly, for 10 minutes.

6 Let cool 10 minutes and then serve.

NET CARBS

8G

SERVES 8

PER SERVING:

CALORIES	488
FAT	39G
PROTEIN	21G
SODIUM	1,300MG
FIBER	2G
CARBOHYDRATES	10G
SUGAR	4G

TIME

PREP TIME:	20 MIN
COOK TIME:	51 MIN

TIPS & OPTIONS

Substitute Italian sausage in link form if desired, just slice the sausage prior to cooking and drain fat.

Add xanthan gum to thicken if desired. Add to soup sparingly, ½ teaspoon xanthan gum at a time, until the desired consistency has been reached. In general, when using xanthan gum, less is more.

TOOTIN' CHILI $ ✗ ◥

NET CARBS

9G

SERVES 10

PER SERVING:

CALORIES	240
FAT	10G
PROTEIN	24G
SODIUM	350MG
FIBER	5G
CARBOHYDRATES	14G
SUGAR	4G

TIME

PREP TIME:	20 MIN
COOK TIME:	50 MIN

TIPS & OPTIONS ⟫

Serve Tootin' Chili with shredded cheese, sour cream, and/or avocado.

To increase fiber, I sometimes add finely diced cooked celery to the base of the Tootin' Chili. *You know I like to add more vegetables wherever I can!*

Chili makes for a great leftover meal. Prepare a double batch to enjoy for three to four days (keep refrigerated).

I hold fond winter memories of eating a giant bowl of chili before becoming a die-hard ketophile. I needed to get this DIRTY, LAZY, KETO–friendly recipe just right in order to cure my hankering for nostalgia. It seems to go best with football on a Sunday afternoon. Canned black soybeans are a delicious keto miracle with only 1g net carbs for ½ cup. More importantly, they taste just like black beans! Fool the eyes and you can dupe the brain too.

2 pounds lean ground turkey

1 medium onion, peeled and diced

1 medium green bell pepper, seeded and chopped

6 cloves garlic, peeled and minced

2 tablespoons tomato paste

1 (28-ounce) can crushed tomatoes

1 (15-ounce) can black soybeans

1 cup water

2 tablespoons chili powder

2 tablespoons paprika

1 tablespoon garlic powder

1 tablespoon onion powder

1 tablespoon ground cumin

½ teaspoon salt

1   In a large pot over medium heat, add turkey and cook 10–15 minutes, stirring regularly until browned. Transfer meat from pot to a large bowl.

2   To the pot, add onion, bell pepper, and garlic. Sauté 3–5 minutes until translucent.

3   Add ground meat, tomato paste, crushed tomatoes, black soybeans, water, and dry spices, stirring regularly.

4   Cover pot and reduce heat. Let simmer 30 minutes until meat is tender.

5   Let cool 10 minutes and then serve.

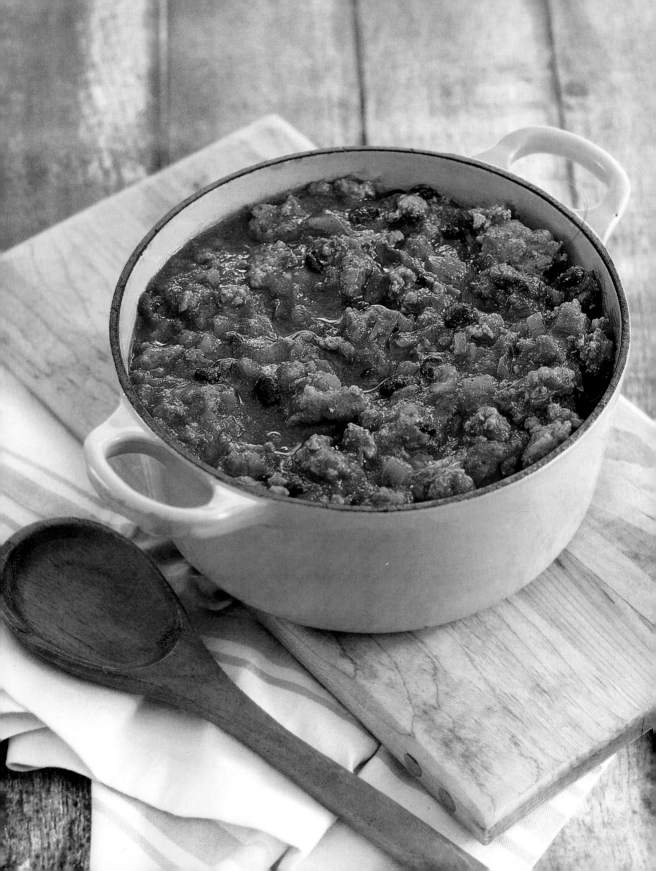

MCDONALD'S CHEESEBURGER SOUP

TIPS & OPTIONS

When served, decorate your soup with typical cheese-burger toppings such as shredded lettuce, a sprinkle of diced onion, sliced pickle, diced tomato, and/or sesame seeds.

Add additional low-carb veggies to your soup portion for variety and healthy fiber.

You can substitute any ground meat of your choice.

My son loves a good burger. The McDonald's cheeseburger is his all-time favorite food! This soup is a budget-friendly, delicious meal that the whole family will enjoy. A package of ground beef stretches a long way when added to soup.

1 pound lean ground beef

3 cups beef broth

4 ounces full-fat cream cheese, cubed

1½ cups shredded Cheddar cheese

4 strips no-sugar-added bacon, cooked and crumbled

¼ cup heavy whipping cream

2 tablespoons unsalted butter

2 tablespoons tomato paste

1 tablespoon yellow mustard

½ teaspoon garlic powder

¼ teaspoon paprika

⅛ teaspoon salt

⅛ teaspoon black pepper

1. In a large pot over medium heat, brown ground beef 5–10 minutes. Drain fat.

2. Stir in broth and cream cheese and cook 3–5 minutes until fully melted. Mix thoroughly.

3. Add in remaining ingredients, stirring 10 minutes until creamy and all cheese is melted.

4. Remove from heat. Let cool 10 minutes and then serve.

LAWN-MOWER SALAD

I'm not a fan of fasting because for me, it feels like punishment. If my weight starts to creep up, I prefer to employ some tried-and-true DIRTY, LAZY, KETO recipes to help me get back under control. This Lawn-Mower Salad is my secret weapon.

3 (12-ounce) bags prewashed broccoli slaw mix

5 (1-gram) packets 0g net carb sweetener

1 tablespoon white vinegar

1 cup full-fat mayonnaise

½ medium red onion, peeled and chopped

1 teaspoon sunflower seeds

In a large mixing bowl, thoroughly mix all ingredients. Serve.

NET CARBS
5G

SERVES 6

PER SERVING:

CALORIES	306
FAT	28G
PROTEIN	5G
SODIUM	283MG
FIBER	6G
CARBOHYDRATES	11G
SUGAR	5G

TIME	
PREP TIME:	5 MIN
COOK TIME:	0 MIN

TIPS & OPTIONS

Add Cheddar cheese or full-fat sour cream to the recipe for added tang.

Mix it up! Instead of slaw mix, try the same recipe using broccoli florets.

Sprinkle bacon bits on top of your salad for added saltiness.

This recipe is one of my favorite "bulk eating" opportunities. Although it technically feeds a family of six, I prefer to eat it all myself. So embarrassing!

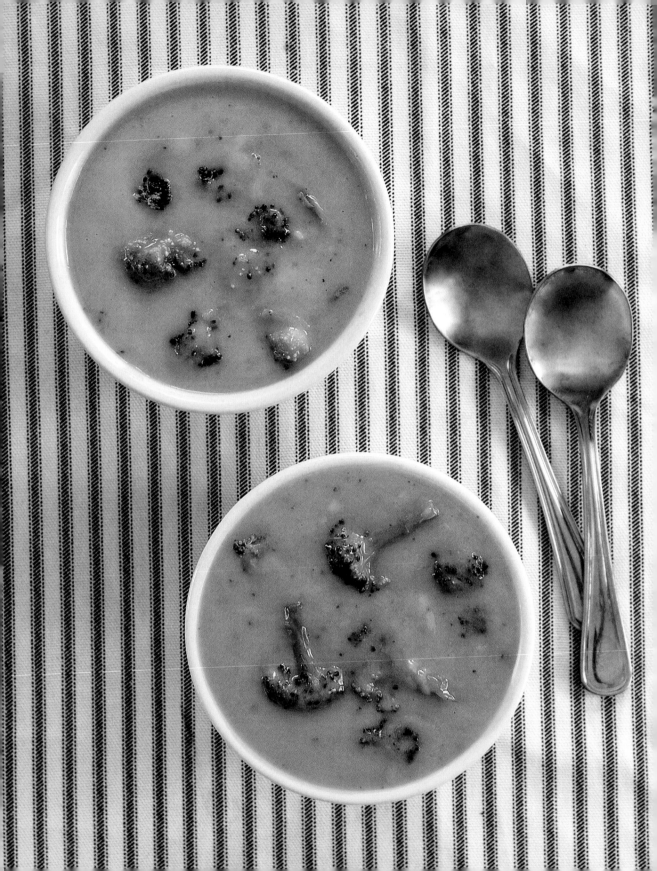

BROC OBAMA CHEESE SOUP $

When my weight starts to creep up, my initial reaction is to go shopping for vegetables. I know myself pretty well, and if I have healthy options in the fridge, I am more likely to make better eating choices. Even though I've kept off 140 pounds for over six years, my weight still fluctuates. **I'm human!** *When you see me pushing a giant pillow of broccoli in my shopping cart, you will know that I've got some work to do and I'm probably getting back on track with Broc Obama Cheese Soup!*

8 cups chicken broth

2 large heads broccoli, chopped into bite-sized florets

1 clove garlic, peeled and minced

¼ cup heavy whipping cream

¼ cup shredded Cheddar cheese

⅛ teaspoon salt

⅛ teaspoon black pepper

1 In a medium pot over medium heat, add broth and bring to boil (about 5 minutes). Add broccoli and garlic. Reduce heat to low, cover pot, and simmer until vegetables are fully softened, about 15 minutes.

2 Remove from heat and blend using a hand immersion blender to desired consistency while still in pot. Leave some chunks of varying sizes for variety.

3 Return pot to medium heat and add cream and cheese. Stir 3–5 minutes until fully blended. Add salt and pepper.

4 Remove from heat, let cool 10 minutes, and serve.

NET CARBS
8G

SERVES 8

PER SERVING:

CALORIES	106
FAT	4G
PROTEIN	7G
SODIUM	1,035MG
FIBER	4G
CARBOHYDRATES	12G
SUGAR	4G

TIME

PREP TIME:	25 MIN
COOK TIME:	25 MIN

TIPS & OPTIONS

Cauliflower can be substituted for the broccoli.

Xanthan gum is an effective low-carb thickener for your soup. Add to soup sparingly, ½ teaspoon xanthan gum at a time, until the desired consistency has been reached. In general, when using xanthan gum, less is more.

LICK-THE-BOWL SALAD DRESSIN' $

TIPS & OPTIONS

I like to pour this salad dressing over an entire bag (or two!) of lettuce, sprinkle with a handful of walnuts, and enjoy while watching TV. I eat the entire bowl by myself, because I'm classy.

Dry mustard is often sold in a strange rectangular yellow tin—I promise this is a normal ingredient sold almost everywhere!

I use either white vinegar or apple cider vinegar as they taste the same to me. No one has convinced me of the difference in health benefits between the two.

I have come to love sesame oil and use it as my "go-to" oil for a secret Asian flavor.

I'm not sure if it was due to cost or preference, but when I was growing up, my dad made his own salad dressing. This family recipe is heavy on the sweet-and-sour flavor, which I just LOVE. I make this in under a minute by shaking the ingredients inside one of those weird "shot glass"–sized Tupperware containers that you've likely never used before (and which drive you crazy since they constantly get caught in your kitchen drawers).

1 teaspoon dry mustard

3 (1-gram) packets 0g net carb sweetener

⅛ teaspoon salt

⅛ teaspoon garlic powder

1 tablespoon white vinegar

4 tablespoons sesame oil

Add all of the ingredients to a 2"-tall (4-ounce) container. Tightly seal lid and shake until blended. Done!

DROP-THE-CHOPSTICK BOWL $ ★ ⬛

When I have a craving for egg rolls, I pull out the skillet to make this Drop-the-Chopstick Bowl. I know intellectually that this probably isn't "real" Chinese food, but smelling soy sauce helps to cure my yen for fried rice and cream cheese wontons. My days of eating fortune cookies, white rice, and sweet-and-sour chicken are long behind me. Having low-carb options like this Drop-the-Chopstick Bowl helps me to stay on track.

2 tablespoons sesame oil

2 cloves garlic, peeled and minced

1 pound lean ground beef

1 (14-ounce) bag coleslaw mix

1 tablespoon sriracha sauce

1 tablespoon white vinegar

2 tablespoons soy sauce

⅛ teaspoon salt

⅛ teaspoon black pepper

1 teaspoon sesame seeds

1 medium green onion, finely chopped

1 In a large skillet over medium heat, heat oil. Add garlic and sauté 1 minute, then add ground beef. Fully cook meat until all pink is gone, approximately 15 minutes. Drain fat.

2 Thoroughly stir in coleslaw mix, sriracha sauce, vinegar, and soy sauce. Cook 10 minutes while stirring until coleslaw is wilted.

3 Season with salt and pepper and garnish with sesame seeds and green onion sprinkled on top.

NET CARBS	
5G	
SERVES 4	
PER SERVING:	
CALORIES	280
FAT	15G
PROTEIN	24G
SODIUM	673MG
FIBER	3G
CARBOHYDRATES	8G
SUGAR	4G

TIME	
PREP TIME:	5 MIN
COOK TIME:	26 MIN

TIPS & OPTIONS

Buy prewashed shredded coleslaw to save time.

Any ground meat can be substituted.

OLIVE GARDEN SALAD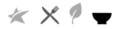

NET CARBS

6G

SERVES 4

PER SERVING:

CALORIES	217
FAT	18G
PROTEIN	4G
SODIUM	948MG
FIBER	2G
CARBOHYDRATES	8G
SUGAR	3G

TIME

PREP TIME:	10 MIN
COOK TIME:	0 MIN

TIPS & OPTIONS

You might be tempted to skip the dressing part of this recipe in lieu of just buying a bottle of the dressing from the restaurant. Hey, I'm with you! I love skipping steps when I can get away with it. Unfortunately, this might be a shortcut that could hurt, not help. The formulation sold at the restaurant contains high-fructose corn syrup as the fourth ingredient; so *not* helpful with weight loss! Make this one yourself.

*As a low-carb eater, I can get pretty depressed eating at Olive Garden. While everyone around me is stuffing their faces with warm breadsticks, I am literally **sitting on my hands**. That is, until the salad arrives. Then I'm all in! Who doesn't love the house salad at Olive Garden? Their unique dressing is what makes the salad so delicious. Since the salad is "unlimited," I will embarrass myself by asking for so many refills that the server gives out dirty looks. Here is my family's re-creation of this spectacular salad. Sorry, but I had to hold the croutons.*

6 cups chopped iceberg lettuce

2 Roma tomatoes, sliced into rounds

¼ cup sliced red onion

1 cup whole pepperoncini

1 cup whole black olives

3 tablespoons olive oil

1 tablespoon red wine vinegar

¼ teaspoon garlic powder

⅛ teaspoon salt

⅛ teaspoon black pepper

⅓ cup grated Parmesan cheese

1 Mix all vegetables and olives in a large salad bowl.

2 In a small bowl, mix oil, vinegar, and spices together.

3 Pour dressing over salad, toss, and top with Parmesan cheese. Serve immediately.

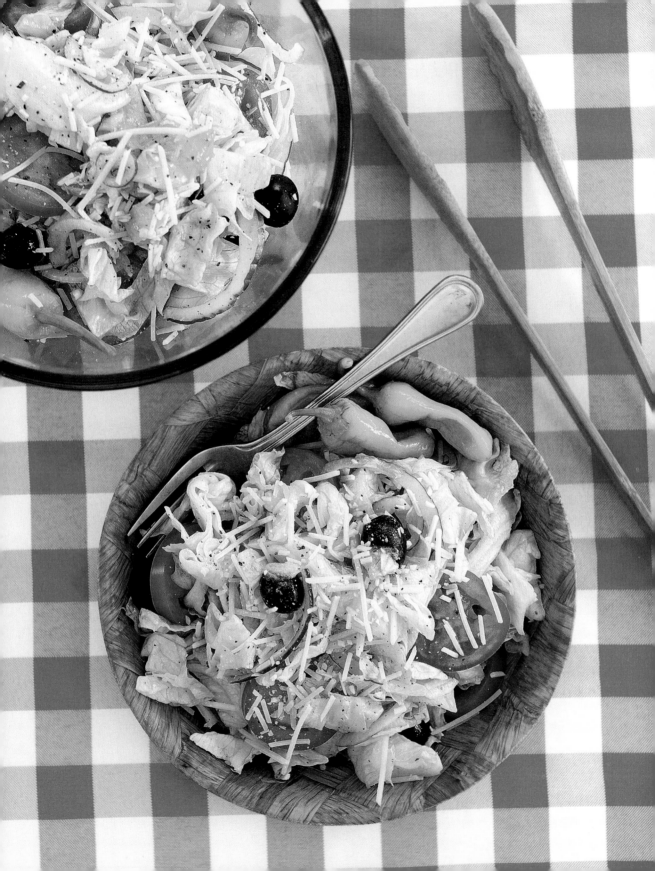

SUMMER TUNA AVOCADO SALAD $

SERVES 4

PER SERVING:

CALORIES	362
FAT	23G
PROTEIN	23G
SODIUM	403MG
FIBER	8G
CARBOHYDRATES	15G
SUGAR	3G

TIME

PREP TIME:	10 MIN
COOK TIME:	0 MIN

TIPS & OPTIONS

For added flair, toss a handful of halved grape tomatoes into this salad.

Dill is an optional substitute for the cilantro.

Since avocados are the "perfect fat" for the keto diet, I am inspired to eat them in as many creative ways as possible. This inexpensive side dish is perfect for a summer barbecue and ensures you have something "safe" to eat at the buffet line.

3 (5-ounce) cans tuna in water, drained and flaked

1 medium cucumber, sliced

3 medium avocados, peeled, pitted, and sliced

1 medium red onion, peeled and sliced

¼ cup finely chopped cilantro

2 tablespoons lemon juice

2 tablespoons olive oil

⅛ teaspoon salt

⅛ teaspoon black pepper

1 In a medium mixing bowl, add drained, flaked tuna.

2 Lightly toss cucumber, avocados, onion, cilantro, lemon juice, and olive oil with tuna. Lightly add salt and pepper at end.

3 Serve immediately.

BIG MAC SALAD $ ★ ✕

A common misconception about DIRTY, LAZY, KETO is that we eat only bacon and cheeseburgers. **So not true!** In fact, we love our vegetables and cheeseburgers equally. This Big Mac Salad is a staple in my household. In addition to loving the Big Mac flavor, I prefer to make meals that can be "reinvented" for the following day. For example, I make turkey tacos one night followed by the Big Mac Salad the next. **Same ingredients, different dinner!** Plus, I find when meals have a fun name like Big Mac Salad, my family is more likely to dig in.

Salad

1 pound lean ground turkey

6 cups chopped iceberg lettuce

1 large pickle, sliced into thin rounds

½ cup diced onion

½ cup diced tomato

⅓ cup shredded Cheddar cheese

1 tablespoon sesame seeds

Special Sauce

¼ cup full-fat mayonnaise

¼ cup no-sugar-added ketchup

1 In a medium skillet over medium heat, cook ground turkey until well done (about 10–15 minutes), stirring regularly. Do not drain fat. Let cool.

2 In a large salad bowl, toss lettuce, pickle, onion, tomato, and shredded cheese.

3 Stir in cooled meat.

4 In a small bowl, mix the sauce ingredients. Add to salad and toss.

5 Sprinkle salad with sesame seeds and serve.

NET CARBS	
6G	

SERVES 4	
PER SERVING:	
CALORIES	347
FAT	23G
PROTEIN	25G
SODIUM	699MG
FIBER	2G
CARBOHYDRATES	8G
SUGAR	5G

TIME	
PREP TIME:	10 MIN
COOK TIME:	15 MIN

◀◀ TIPS & OPTIONS

Picky Eaters Method: Prepare individual plates of lettuce and miniature bowls of toppings and set up like a buffet. Family members can pick and choose which toppings they would like and build their own custom salads.

You may substitute ground beef for this recipe (drain the fat).

Sprinkle light amounts of tomato on your portion of the Big Mac Salad and remember: Tomatoes are higher in carbs.

Buy bagged salad mix to save time or wash/cut up your own head of preferred lettuce.

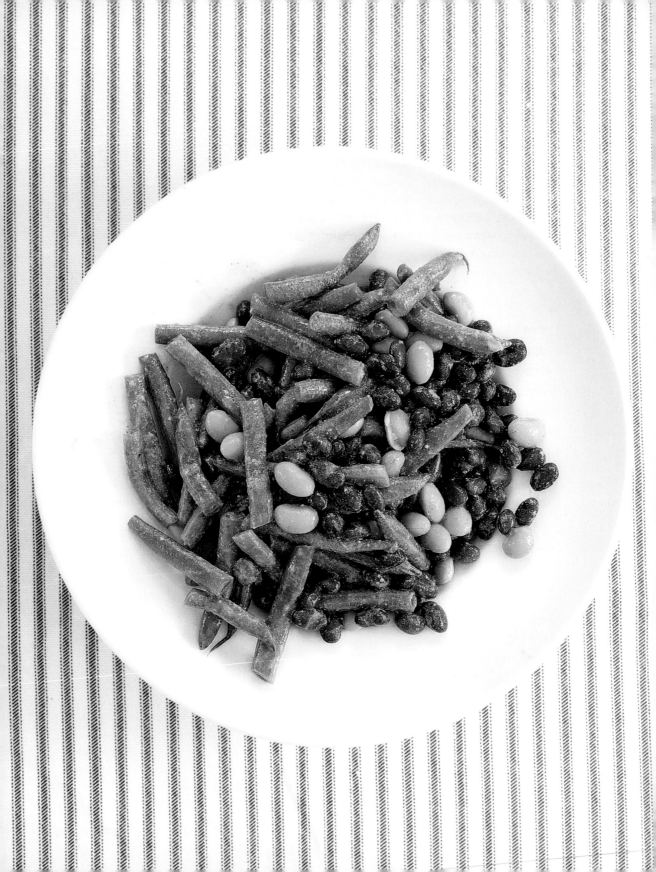

VINTAGE THREE BEAN SALAD

*When I started the DIRTY, LAZY, KETO way of eating, I thought I was saying goodbye to beans forever. I wanted to re-create my mother's 1950s-era Three Bean Salad favorite, but without all the carbs. This proved challenging until I discovered black soybeans as an alternative ingredient. Whenever I eat Vintage Three Bean Salad, I am transported back in time to an era when ladies hosted luncheons while wearing girdles and white gloves. Maybe **that's why** the women were so skinny back then?*

3 cups fresh green beans, trimmed and cut into 2" lengths

½ cup shelled soybeans (edamame), cooked

1 cup black soybeans

3 tablespoons olive oil

2 tablespoons apple cider vinegar

1 tablespoon lemon juice

1 teaspoon spicy mustard

1 clove garlic, peeled and minced

2 tablespoons dried basil, or chopped fresh

⅛ teaspoon salt

⅛ teaspoon black pepper

1   In a medium microwave-safe bowl, microwave raw green beans 4 minutes with ¼ cup water. Drain water and let cool.

2   In a medium mixing bowl, combine green beans with other two beans.

3   In a small bowl, whisk remaining ingredients to make dressing.

4   Pour dressing over beans and lightly toss.

5   If desired, chill before serving.

NET CARBS	
6G	
SERVES 4	
PER SERVING:	
CALORIES	204
FAT	14G
PROTEIN	10G
SODIUM	111MG
FIBER	7G
CARBOHYDRATES	13G
SUGAR	3G

TIME	
PREP TIME:	15 MIN
COOK TIME:	4 MIN

TIPS & OPTIONS

Black soybeans can be hard to find. At this time, I have seen them available only online.

For added bulk, crunch, and flavor, consider the addition of a sturdy vegetable like finely chopped cucumber or celery.

CHAPTER 5

SNACKS

"Hanger" anxiety. Have you ever listened to Jim Gaffigan's comedy routine about people on vacation, going from one meal to the next? "Why don't we eat something, and then we'll go get something to eat?" I can't do his humor justice, but I can attest that Gaffigan's jokes get right to the point. I am constantly eating, and when I put down the fork, I start thinking about what to eat next (and I'm not even on vacation!).

I suffer from hunger anxiety. I'm being honest, here, however irrational it may sound. I actually fear the consequences of a rumbling stomach. I am terrified that in an extreme state of "hanger," I will start making poor eating choices, and subsequently gain all of my weight back in one sitting. (May I remind you that this is my *irrational fear?*) To avoid facing this dire situation, I have developed a habit of constantly snacking.

Part of the reason I have been so successful with losing 140 pounds and keeping it off for six years is that I lean into my idiosyncrasies. I stopped judging myself long ago. I embrace my quirkiness and even celebrate my uniqueness. I am a frequent snacker! I AM AFRAID OF HUNGER!

You might be laughing now, but if we get trapped in a broken elevator together, rest assured I'll be pulling out a Ziploc bag of chicken breast and room-temperature cheese sticks.

DRAGON TAIL JALAPEÑO POPPAHS

NET CARBS
4G

SERVES 8

PER SERVING:

CALORIES	137
FAT	11G
PROTEIN	3G
SODIUM	406MG
FIBER	0G
CARBOHYDRATES	4G
SUGAR	3G

TIME

PREP TIME:	15 MIN
COOK TIME:	19MIN

TIPS & OPTIONS

Wrap each jalapeño half with a half strip of bacon (either turkey or pork). Make sure to slice the bacon in half lengthwise so the skinny slice of bacon wraps around the jalapeño half several times, ensuring it stays secure without a toothpick.

Very Important Wear food-grade gloves during the handling of the cut jalapeños! Trust me, if you don't wear gloves or don't wash your hands thoroughly with dish soap and a scrub brush before rubbing your eyes or touching any other "sensitive" areas, you will be in a world of hurt.

This has to be the recipe I am most excited to share with you. Dragon Tail Jalapeño Poppahs involve two aspects of food that I love: warm, gooey cheese and spicy peppers. For a classier presentation, keep the stem attached to one of the halves during preparation. Now you have a handy-dandy handle for your poppah!

8 (2") jalapeños, halved, seeded, and deveined

4 ounces full-fat cream cheese, softened

¼ cup full-fat mayonnaise

1 (1-ounce) package ranch powder seasoning mix

½ cup shredded Cheddar cheese

1   Preheat oven to 375°F. Line a baking sheet with parchment paper.

2   In a medium microwave-safe bowl, microwave peppers with ¼ cup water for 3 minutes to soften. Drain and let cool.

3   Line up peppers on baking sheet, cut-side up.

4   In a separate medium microwave-safe bowl, add cream cheese, mayonnaise, ranch powder, and shredded cheese. Microwave for 30 seconds and stir. Microwave another 15 seconds and stir.

5   Carefully scoop mixture into sandwich-sized bag. Snip off one corner to make a hole (the width of a pencil).

6   Using makeshift pastry bag, fill jalapeño halves evenly with mixture.

7   Bake 15 minutes until peppers are fully softened and cheese is golden brown.

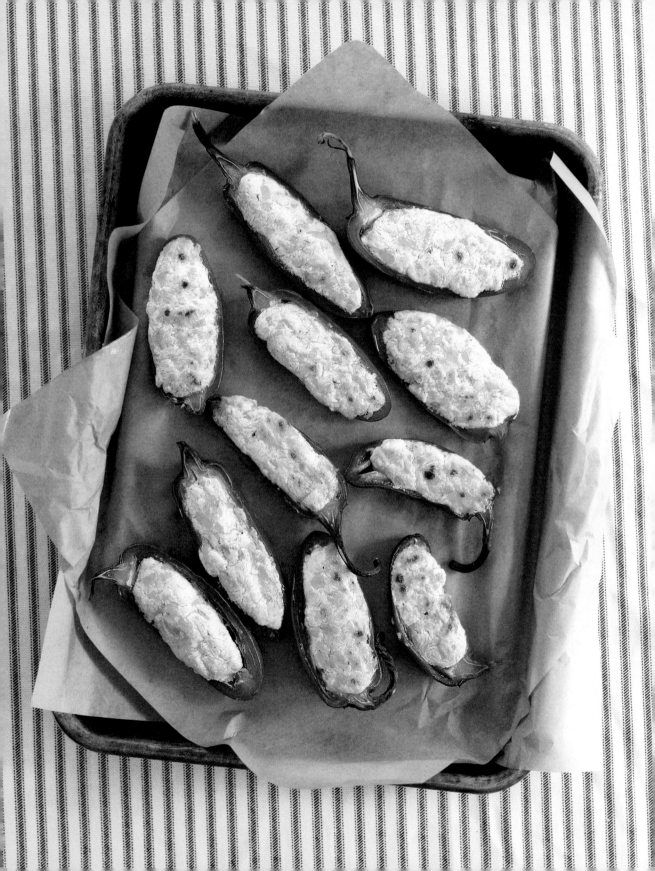

CUBED TOFU FRIES $

Just like my inability to solve a Rubik's Cube, I have yet to find a satisfying French fry alternative. Like rearranging all the stickers to beat the cube, I am willing to pull out all of the stops to accomplish my goal of creating a winning recipe. As crazy as it sounds, Cubed Tofu Fries have just enough salt and fat to fool my brain.

1 (12-ounce) package extra-firm tofu

2 tablespoons sesame oil

⅛ teaspoon salt, divided

⅛ teaspoon black pepper, divided

⅛ teaspoon creole seasoning, divided

1 Remove tofu from packaging and wrap in paper towel. Set on a clean plate. Place a second plate on top and put a 3- to 5-pound weight on top. Let sit 20 minutes. Drain excess water.

2 Unwrap tofu and slice into small cubes no larger than ½" square (a little larger than sugar cubes).

3 In a large skillet over medium heat, heat oil.

4 Combine salt, pepper, and creole seasoning in a small bowl. Sprinkle one-third of spice mixture evenly into skillet and add tofu evenly.

5 Sprinkle one-third of spices on top and let fry 5 minutes on each side, flipping three times (for the four sides), browning all four sides.

6 Dust tofu with remaining spice mixture.

7 Remove from heat. Enjoy while hot!

NET CARBS

0G

SERVES 4

PER SERVING:

CALORIES	119
FAT	10G
PROTEIN	7G
SODIUM	126MG
FIBER	1G
CARBOHYDRATES	1G
SUGAR	1G

TIME

PREP TIME:	25 MIN
COOK TIME:	20 MIN

TIPS & OPTIONS

Try to get the firm or extra-firm tofu that is in a plastic tray and packaged with water. The type that is in the cardboard block is a lot more moist, and it is harder to fry while keeping its shape.

Using well-drained, extra-firm tofu helps the cubes maintain their shape during the cooking process. Otherwise, the tofu shapes will crumble when stirred, resulting in a scrambled egg–style mess (that still tastes great but isn't as pretty).

I once varied my recipe to season the tofu with cinnamon and Splenda. The result was so delicious that I ended up eating *two* full blocks of tofu in one sitting.

SARAH'S EXPERT CRACKERS

DIRTY, LAZY, KETO: Recipes, Inspiration, & Support Facebook group member Sarah (age fifty-six) has lost over a hundred pounds (and has kept it off four years) by following a low-carb lifestyle. Her expert cracker recipe beats anything I've ever tried. Sarah is the "real deal" in the kitchen!

1 cup blanched almond flour

2 tablespoons hemp hearts

2 tablespoons flaxseed meal

2 tablespoons psyllium husk powder

2 tablespoons chia seeds

2 tablespoons shelled pumpkin seeds

2 tablespoons Everything and More seasoning

½ tablespoon salt

1½ cups water

1 squirt liquid stevia

1 Preheat oven to 350°F.

2 In a medium mixing bowl, combine dry ingredients.

3 Add water and liquid stevia and mix together until a thick dough is formed.

4 Place dough between two pieces of parchment paper and roll out to desired cracker thickness.

5 Remove top piece of parchment paper and use a pizza cutter to cut dough into desired cracker shapes.

6 While cracker shapes are still on bottom piece of parchment paper, put on a baking sheet and into oven.

7 Bake 30–40 minutes until centers of crackers are hard.

8 Let cool 5 minutes, then serve.

NET CARBS

5G

SERVES 10

PER SERVING:

CALORIES	111
FAT	6G
PROTEIN	5G
SODIUM	541MG
FIBER	2G
CARBOHYDRATES	7G
SUGAR	1G

TIME

PREP TIME:	15 MIN
COOK TIME:	40 MIN

TIPS & OPTIONS

Pair this cracker recipe with El Presidente Guac or Cucumber Sallllllllsaaaaa to serve at your next party (see recipes in this chapter).

Any powdered 0g net carb sweetener can be switched with the liquid stevia.

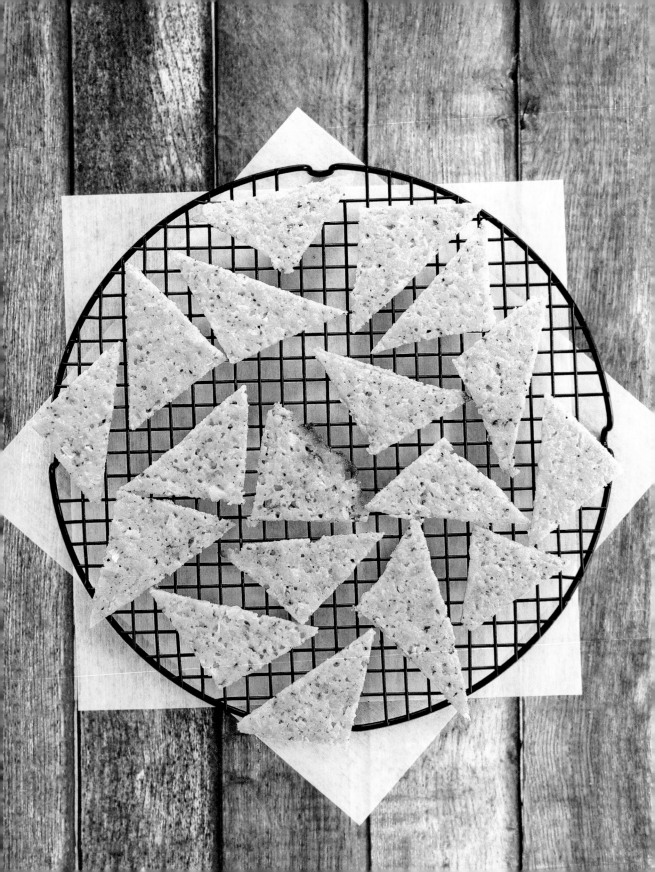

COOL RANCH DORITO CRACKERS

Sometimes when you are on the couch watching TV, you harken back to the old days when cheese and crackers or a bag of chips was your trusty companion. Yes, you can buy a bag of those expensive protein chips and break the bank, or you can easily make homemade Cool Ranch Dorito Crackers! In moderation, cheese is DIRTY, LAZY, KETO–friendly; this simple cracker recipe may fill the chip void.

2 cups riced cauliflower, uncooked

1½ cups grated Parmesan cheese

2 teaspoons ranch seasoning powder

⅛ teaspoon salt

⅛ teaspoon black pepper

1 Preheat oven to 375°F.

2 In a medium microwave-safe bowl, microwave riced cauliflower 1 minute. Stir and microwave 1 more minute.

3 Let cool and scoop cauliflower onto a clean dish towel. Squeeze out excess water.

4 Return to bowl and add Parmesan, ranch seasoning, salt, and pepper. Mix thoroughly until moist dough is formed.

5 Place the dough on a large piece of parchment paper. Then place a second piece of parchment paper on top of the dough. Use a rolling pin to flatten the dough to the thickness of a Dorito.

6 After the dough is rolled to the desired thickness, remove the top piece of parchment paper and use a pizza cutter to cut the dough into triangle shapes that are roughly the size of Doritos.

7 Transfer the parchment paper with the cut crackers to a baking sheet. Leave enough space between each cracker so they cook evenly and won't stick to nearby crackers during baking.

8 Bake 25–35 minutes until golden brown.

9 Let cool and serve.

NET CARBS

4G

SERVES 7

PER SERVING:

CALORIES	98
FAT	5G
PROTEIN	7G
SODIUM	510MG
FIBER	1G
CARBOHYDRATES	5G
SUGAR	1G

TIME

PREP TIME:	15 MIN
COOK TIME:	37 MIN

TIPS & OPTIONS

Make sure your final product is crispy and dry. *No one likes soggy crackers!*

Pair these crackers with one of the many low-carb dips included in this cookbook.

CHIPPED ARTICHOKES

NET CARBS

3G

SERVES 4

PER SERVING:

CALORIES	219
FAT	20G
PROTEIN	2G
SODIUM	497MG
FIBER	5G
CARBOHYDRATES	8G
SUGAR	1G

TIME

PREP TIME:	5 MIN
COOK TIME:	35 MIN

TIPS & OPTIONS ≫

Prepare the artichoke by trimming at least the top inch off, cutting the artichoke nearly in half. This allows the steam to reach inside.

Feel free to cut artichokes vertically in half (at the stem) to speed up the steaming process.

Remove the tough outer part of the stem with a peeler.

When you get to the last of the outer leaves, use a spoon to scrape out the tiny spindly baby leaves/needles from the artichoke heart. Be careful to remove all of these needles as they are a choking hazard.

Living in California, I have year-round access to an abundance of fresh produce. In fact, the artichoke capital of the world is advertised to be in Castroville, California—not too far from where I live. I'm able to enjoy artichoke "chip alternatives" year-round for a reasonable price. I eat artichokes like I used to snack on chips. Even better, I dip each leaf into a bath of full-fat mayonnaise mixed with lemon juice and salt. As someone who avoided mayo for their entire life prior to DIRTY, LAZY, KETO, I just can't get enough of the stuff now.

½ teaspoon salt, divided

2 large artichokes, trimmed

2 tablespoons lemon juice

½ cup full-fat mayonnaise

1   In a large pot, prepare 1" water with ¼ teaspoon salt.

2   Put artichokes in a steamer basket inside pot, stem-side up, and cover pot. When boiling starts, reduce heat to medium-low and leave untouched 25 minutes.

3   Test to see if done by pulling off outer leaf using tongs. If it doesn't come off easily, add additional water to pot and steam 5–10 more minutes. Let cool.

4   Serve with dip made by combining lemon juice, mayonnaise, and remaining salt.

ROAD TRIP RED PEPPER EDAMAME

Even my "picky-eater" son loves to snack on lightly salted edamame. I prefer this "grown-up" version of soybeans, brought alive with spicy red pepper flakes! I adapt this recipe to feed us both. Edamame is a perfect road trip snack. Instead of eating chips, try a salty bag of Road Trip Red Pepper Edamame during your travels.

2 cups frozen raw edamame in the shell

1 tablespoon peanut oil

2 cloves garlic, peeled and minced

⅛ teaspoon salt

½ teaspoon red pepper flakes

1   In a medium microwave-safe bowl with ½ cup water, microwave edamame 4–5 minutes.

2   In a medium saucepan over medium heat, add peanut oil. Add minced garlic and salt. Stir 3–5 minutes to soften garlic.

3   Add edamame and stir 2–3 minutes until well heated and coated. Turn off heat and cover saucepan to steam edamame for 5 additional minutes.

4   Remove lid. Add red pepper flakes and toss to coat.

5   Serve immediately for best results.

NET CARBS	
3G	

SERVES 4	
PER SERVING:	
CALORIES	131
FAT	7G
PROTEIN	10G
SODIUM	87MG
FIBER	6G
CARBOHYDRATES	9G
SUGAR	1G

TIME	
PREP TIME:	1 MIN
COOK TIME:	18 MIN

TIPS & OPTIONS

I often buy frozen edamame. It's cheaper and available year-round.

Is this your first time eating edamame? Do not eat the outside shell! Instead, pinch the bean pod with your teeth and slide the pod until a slick little bean pops out into your mouth. Soybeans are a snack (and fun activity) all in one.

STUFFED PARTY SHROOMS $ ◉

TIPS & OPTIONS 》》

Large portabella mushrooms also work well. They are easier to prepare since there will be fewer of them. Bake them longer due to their size.

For added variety, try adding chopped jalapeño, crab-meat, or a different cheese to your stuffed mushrooms.

Stuffed Party Shrooms are a delicacy worth the prep work. Similar to making Devilish Eggs (see recipe in this chapter), this appetizer involves a lot of time at the kitchen sink. The creepiest part of this recipe involves removing the gills from the mushrooms. What exactly is all of that matter underneath the mushroom cap? Whether you prepare Stuffed Party Shrooms for a special gathering of guests, or make a platter to enjoy by yourself while watching TV, stuffed mushrooms are a fantastic keto-friendly snack.

12 large whole mushrooms, approximately 2" wide

2 tablespoons unsalted butter

8 ounces cooked no-sugar-added bacon, crumbled (approximately 8 strips)

7 ounces full-fat cream cheese, softened

½ cup full-fat mayonnaise

1 medium green onion, finely chopped

1 teaspoon paprika

⅛ teaspoon salt

⅛ teaspoon black pepper

1   Preheat oven to 400°F. Line a baking sheet with parchment paper.

2   Remove mushroom stems from caps, being very careful not to break edges of cap, and scrape out the black gills if the mushroom is mature enough for the gills to be visible. Chop the trimmed stem pieces finely.

3   In a small frying pan over medium heat, fry mushroom trimmings with butter for 3 minutes until soft.

4   Place caps on baking sheet, rounded-side down.

5   In a medium bowl, combine fried mushroom trimmings with remaining ingredients. Scoop the mixture evenly into the caps.

6   Bake 20 minutes until filling bubbles and turns golden brown.

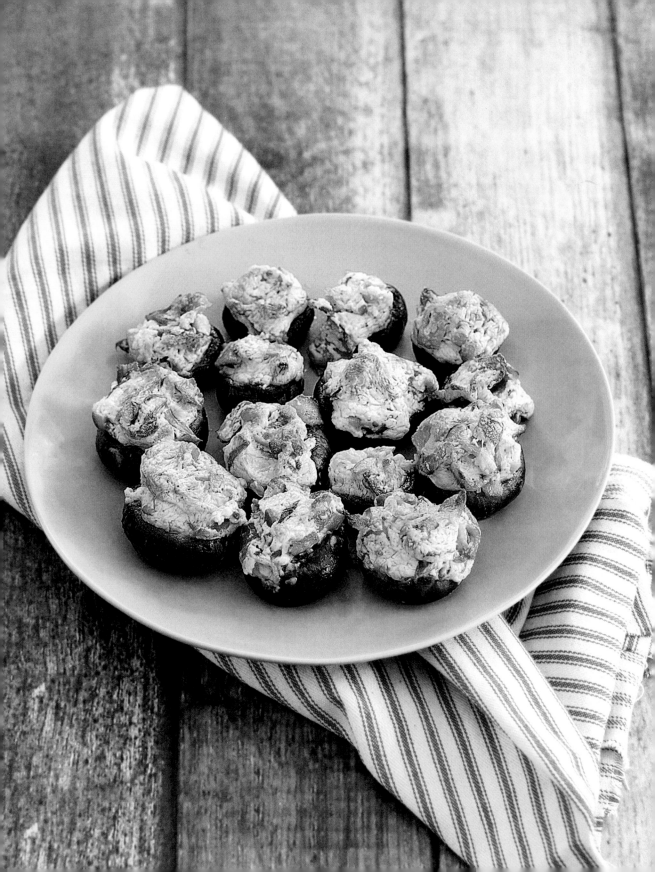

CLASSY CRUDITÉS AND DIP

NET CARBS

6G

SERVES 8

PER SERVING:

CALORIES	146
FAT	10G
PROTEIN	4G
SODIUM	88MG
FIBER	3G
CARBOHYDRATES	9G
SUGAR	5G

TIME

PREP TIME:	15 MIN
COOK TIME:	0 MIN

TIPS & OPTIONS ≫

Mix and match the in-season vegetables you already have.

The dip can be "amped up" with a little creole seasoning (salt, pepper, chili powder, cayenne, and garlic powder), which adds color and heat.

Save time and skip the dip-making step altogether! Pour ranch salad dressing into a bowl for dipping. *I won't tell.*

Add olives, cubed cheese, and even salami to your crudités platter for a superb appetizer.

You know what's best about crudités and dip? Most grocery stores sell assorted premade vegetable platters at a reasonable price. If washing and prepping vegetables takes up too much of your time, and you suspect buying a platter will help you to eat healthier, I say skip that step and toss a premade platter into your grocery cart! Like buying a jar of premade pesto sauce, sometimes spending a little extra money for convenience is worth it. Crudités and dip platters are perfect for holidays and get-togethers. It's a "safe food" for you to eat in excess, and party guests will appreciate the healthy gesture among a sea of high-carb buffet options.

Vegetables

1 cup whole cherry tomatoes

1 cup green beans, trimmed

2 cups broccoli florets

2 cups cauliflower florets

1 bunch asparagus, trimmed

1 large green bell pepper, seeded and chopped

Sour Cream Dip

2 cups full-fat sour cream

3 tablespoons dry chives

1 tablespoon lemon juice

½ cup dried parsley

½ teaspoon garlic powder

⅛ teaspoon salt

⅛ teaspoon black pepper

1 Cut vegetables into bite-sized uniform pieces. Arrange in like groups around outside edge of a large serving platter, leaving room in middle for dip.

2 Make dip by combining dip ingredients in a medium-sized decorative bowl and mixing well.

3 Place dip bowl in the center of platter and serve.

DEVILISH EGGS $ ◉ ✕ 🌱

Deviled eggs are a proven crowd-pleaser! But I used to avoid making these Devilish Eggs because I had so much trouble peeling the eggs. The shells would stick to the egg whites, and I would end up losing half of the product trying to get it unglued. It wasn't until I discovered the miracle of making hard-boiled eggs in the pressure cooker that I revisited this beloved recipe. Now, the egg shells peel off so easily—"like butta!" Because of the pressure cooker, I now make Devilish Eggs on a regular basis. They're inexpensive, healthy, and popular with my guests.

6 large eggs

3 tablespoons full-fat mayonnaise

1 teaspoon plain white vinegar

1 teaspoon spicy mustard

⅛ teaspoon salt

⅛ teaspoon black pepper

⅛ teaspoon ground cayenne

⅛ teaspoon paprika

NET CARBS	
1G	

SERVES 6	

PER SERVING:

CALORIES	125
FAT	9G
PROTEIN	6G
SODIUM	164MG
FIBER	0G
CARBOHYDRATES	1G
SUGAR	1G

TIME	
PREP TIME:	10 MIN
COOK TIME:	9 MIN

1 Preferred Method: Hard-boil eggs using a steamer basket in the Instant Pot® on high pressure for 9 minutes. Release pressure and remove eggs.

2 Alternate Method: Place eggs in a large pot. Cover with water by 1". Cover with a lid and place the pot over high heat until it reaches a boil. Turn off heat, leave covered, and let it sit for 13 minutes. Then, remove the eggs from the pan, place them in an ice water bath, and let them cool 5 minutes.

3 When cooled, peel eggs and slice in half lengthwise. Place yolks in a medium bowl.

4 Mash and mix yolks with mayonnaise, vinegar, mustard, salt, and black pepper.

5 Scrape mixture into a sandwich-sized plastic bag and snip off one corner, making a hole about the width of a pencil. Use makeshift pastry bag to fill egg white halves with yolk mixture.

6 Garnish Devilish Eggs with cayenne and paprika (mostly for color) and serve.

《 TIPS & OPTIONS

I've tried following the urban legend about sprinkling baking soda into the boiling water to help make the eggs easier to peel, but did not have much success.

On Halloween, when my party guests are shoving candy into their mouths, I am eating Devilish Eggs. By adding a slice of black olive to the top, this cute appetizer turns into a scary "eyeball." If you have red food coloring on hand, you can "draw" bloodshot lines on the white egg part using a toothpick.

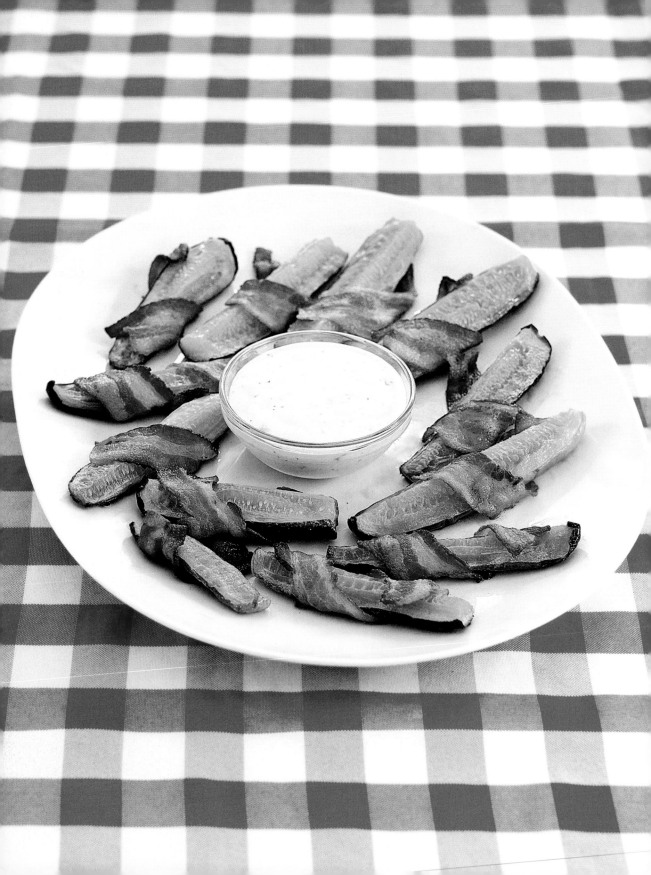

HANGOVER BACON-WRAPPED PICKLES

Losing weight with DIRTY, LAZY, KETO leads to salt cravings. It's part of the process! Hangover Bacon-Wrapped Pickles are the perfect salty snack. After you make a batch, be sure to store the jar of leftover pickle juice in the fridge. In addition to preventing a hangover, pickle juice works wonders to prevent the mythical "keto flu."

3 large pickles

6 strips uncooked no-sugar-added bacon, cut in half lengthwise

¼ cup ranch dressing

1 Preheat oven to 425°F. Line a baking sheet with foil.

2 Quarter each pickle lengthwise (yielding twelve spears).

3 Wrap each spear with a half strip bacon. Place on baking sheet.

4 Bake 20 minutes or until crispy, flipping at the midpoint.

5 Serve your crispy bacon-wrapped pickles while still hot with a side of the ranch dipping sauce.

NET CARBS	
2G	

SERVES 4	
PER SERVING:	
CALORIES	96
FAT	6G
PROTEIN	6G
SODIUM	1,117MG
FIBER	1G
CARBOHYDRATES	3G
SUGAR	1G

TIME	
PREP TIME:	5 MIN
COOK TIME:	20 MIN

TIPS & OPTIONS

Use toothpicks (soaked in water) to pin the bacon. Soaking the toothpicks ahead of time prevents them from burning in the oven.

If you're feeding a hesitant crowd, make smaller portions by dicing and wrapping smaller "bites" of pickles.

SNAPPY BACON ASPARAGUS

TIPS & OPTIONS

Soak toothpicks in water to prevent them from blackening during the cooking process.

Asparagus wrapped in no-sugar-added pork bacon cooks quickly on the grill because of the high fat content. Keep the temperature at medium-low heat to ensure the asparagus (not just the bacon), has time to thoroughly cook.

If you use turkey bacon, like I usually do, brush additional olive oil onto each wrapped asparagus bunch to help "crisp" the bacon.

Whether fried, cooked in the toaster oven, or grilled on a barbecue, bacon-wrapped asparagus is always a hit with my family. My kids love to help assemble these "French fry substitutes." Years ago, I offered up a convincing tale that asparagus turns your pee green! (This fact has yet to be verified in my household, but the story continues to encourage asparagus eating from my little ones.)

24 asparagus spears

6 strips no-sugar-added bacon, uncooked

2 tablespoons olive oil

⅛ teaspoon salt

1 My favorite part of preparing asparagus is the SNAP. Grab the "nonpointed" end of stalk and bend until it breaks. This usually happens about an inch from the end with the cut. Now, line up asparagus and cut entire bunch at "snapping" point, making all of your stalks uniform in length. Fancy, right?

2 On a microwave-safe plate, microwave asparagus 2 minutes to soften. Let cool 5 minutes.

3 Lay strip of bacon on a cutting board at 45-degree angle. Lay four asparagus spears centered on bacon in an "up and down" position.

4 Pick up bacon and asparagus where they meet and wrap two ends of bacon around asparagus in opposite directions.

5 Wrap bacon tightly and secure, pinning bacon to asparagus at ends with toothpicks. Don't worry if bacon doesn't cover entire spears.

6 Brush asparagus with olive oil and sprinkle with salt.

7 Heat a medium nonstick skillet over medium heat. Cook asparagus/bacon 3–5 minutes per side while turning to cook thoroughly. Continue flipping until bacon is brown and crispy.

CUCUMBER SALLLLLLLLSAAAAA $

As a kid of the 1990s, one of my favorite Seinfeld *episodes was the one when Jerry talked about his favorite word, Sallllllllsaaaaa. He just liked saying it aloud. Try it! This recipe is cool and refreshing. I recommend serving Cucumber Sallllllllsaaaaa atop grilled whitefish. You can pretend you are on an exotic Caribbean vacation at a Mexican restaurant (minus the carbolicious basket of chips)!*

2 medium cucumbers

2 medium tomatoes

4 medium jalapeño peppers, deveined, seeded, and finely chopped

½ medium red onion, peeled and chopped

1 clove garlic, peeled and minced

2 tablespoons lime juice

2 teaspoons dried parsley

2 teaspoons finely chopped cilantro

½ teaspoon salt

1. Finely chop or pulse cucumbers and tomatoes separately in a food processor to desired consistency.

2. Add to a large mixing bowl along with rest of ingredients and mix thoroughly. Serve.

NET CARBS	
5G	

SERVES 8

PER SERVING:

CALORIES	23
FAT	0G
PROTEIN	1G
SODIUM	149MG
FIBER	1G
CARBOHYDRATES	6G
SUGAR	3G

TIME

PREP TIME:	10 MIN
COOK TIME:	0 MIN

TIPS & OPTIONS

For variety, add sliced avocado or even feta cheese to your salsa.

BUFFALO BILL'S CHICKEN DIP

NET CARBS

5G

SERVES 10

PER SERVING:

CALORIES	538
FAT	43G
PROTEIN	25G
SODIUM	1,236MG
FIBER	0G
CARBOHYDRATES	5G
SUGAR	2G

TIME

PREP TIME:	15 MIN
COOK TIME:	30 MIN

TIPS & OPTIONS

This dip is best served warm.

Make sure that you use the plain buffalo wing sauce, not one that is creamy or sweet.

Raw cucumbers, celery, broccoli, and cauliflower make excellent choices for "dippers."

Buffalo Bill's Chicken Dip is great for get-togethers. It's a bit spicy, so it will probably be better suited for an adult crowd. The ranch powdered seasoning mix is the secret ingredient. When this is on sale, I stock up. Don't laugh, but I currently have about fifty packets in my pantry right now. Between this dish and my Dragon Tail Jalapeño Poppahs recipe in this chapter, I use this secret ingredient quite a bit!

2 (4.2-ounce) chicken breasts from cooked rotisserie chicken

1 (8-ounce) package full-fat cream cheese, softened

2 cups shredded whole milk mozzarella cheese

1 cup shredded Cheddar cheese

1 (1-ounce) package ranch powder seasoning mix

1 cup full-fat mayonnaise

1 cup full-fat sour cream

½ cup finely chopped green onion

¼ cup buffalo wing sauce

1 teaspoon garlic powder

½ pound no-sugar-added bacon, cooked and crumbled

1 Preheat oven to 350°F. Grease a 2-quart (8" × 8") baking dish.

2 In a small bowl, finely shred chicken.

3 Combine chicken with remaining ingredients, except bacon, in baking dish, stirring to mix well.

4 Bake 25–30 minutes; stop when bubbling and browned on top.

5 Take out of the oven and stir again to mix all the melted ingredients. Top with the crumbled bacon. Serve immediately.

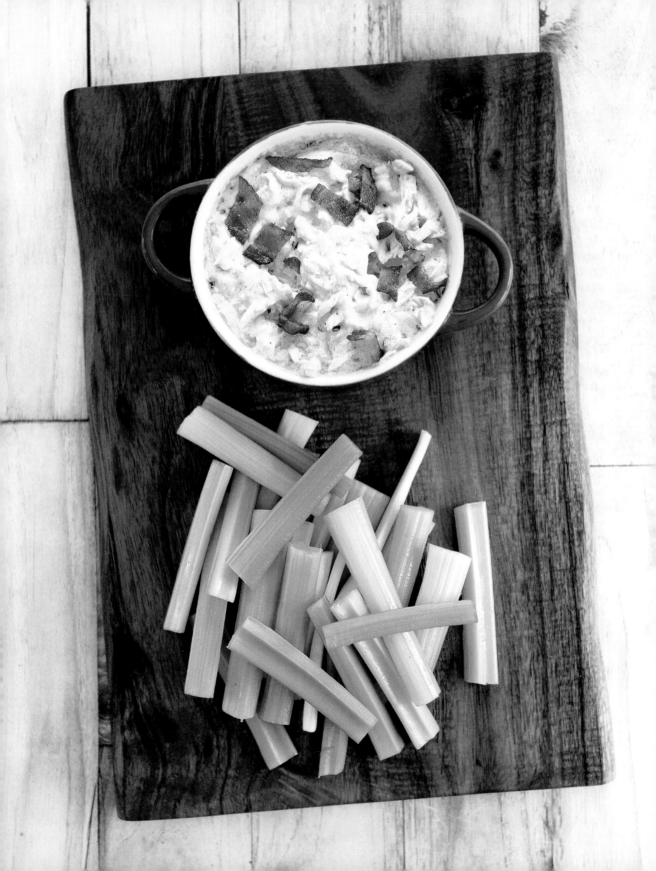

EL PRESIDENTE GUAC

NET CARBS

5G

SERVES 4

PER SERVING:

CALORIES	131
FAT	9G
PROTEIN	2G
SODIUM	83MG
FIBER	5G
CARBOHYDRATES	10G
SUGAR	1G

TIME

PREP TIME:	10 MIN
COOK TIME:	0 MIN

TIPS & OPTIONS »

I prefer to use Roma tomatoes in my guac because they are firmer and are easier to slice.

To increase the heat, add finely chopped jalapeños and onion. Remember to vein and seed your jalapeños, or you will be in for a surprise!

To speed up the ripening process of your avocados, place them in a paper bag with a banana. The fruits will help oxidize each other.

Avocados symbolize the keto community. They taste delicious and offer a quick source of healthy fats. This simple guacamole recipe is good enough to serve el presidente!

2 large avocados, peeled and pitted

1 tablespoon garlic powder

1 tablespoon onion powder

⅛ teaspoon salt

⅛ teaspoon chili powder

4 tablespoons finely chopped cilantro

1 Roma tomato, finely chopped

4 teaspoons lime juice

1. In a medium bowl, mash avocados and combine with dry spices.

2. Add cilantro, tomato, and lime juice and mix again. Serve.

CHAPTER 6

BREADS, PASTA, AND PIZZA

"Weirdoughs" and "impastas." Whether you are suffering from a hangover (did I just say that?) or returning from a two-day church retreat, there is a feeling of warmth and completeness that one experiences when they sit down to a meal composed of comfort food that includes bread, pasta, or pizza. There is no reason you can't continue to enjoy traditional comfort food recipes on a regular basis. My favorite recipes here have been "tweaked" to reduce carbohydrate levels while maintaining flavor.

People often ask me if my family is onboard with the DIRTY, LAZY, KETO lifestyle. They wonder if I make multiple meals every night to meet everyone's dietary preferences. Here is my quick answer: NOPE! My son likes to repeatedly swing open the fridge doors while shouting, "THERE IS NOTHING TO EAT!" I translate his frustration to mean, "There is no junk food here!" *That's correct, my love.*

I prepare hearty dinners that everyone in my family can enjoy. There is nothing "bad" about a DIRTY, LAZY, KETO dish. As you see here, there are no weird or scary ingredients. That's not to say I'm a "carb hater" toward the rest of my non-keto family members. They are welcome to enjoy pasta, rice, tortillas, potatoes, and more to accompany the meal that I prepared. *My only request* is that they fix that part themselves. Is that so outrageous? I don't feel bad, at all, for asking my kids to boil a pot of water and set a timer.

If your family really wants a side of rice, can't they figure out how to make it themselves?

Change is NOT easy. You are challenging the family's current belief system about food. You might even be scaring your family. Inside, they might feel worried about why you're trying to change. They fear, "Are we not enough? Does she want something MORE?"

> Folks like the idea of you becoming healthier, but not when it means their beloved Chips Ahoys are missing from the pantry.

The answer, if you want to get out in front of this, is YES! *Yes, you do want something more for yourself!* Don't be afraid to admit this. You want your health back. You want your body back. You want to be the partner, parent, or child you dreamed of becoming. The DIRTY, LAZY, KETO way of life involves a massive transformation of existing norms in your household, and that, my friend, takes leadership and courage. If the only person you hear this from is me, let me say it loudly: I'm proud of you!

For now, however, let's focus on comfort food. My collection of bread, pasta, and pizza recipes will warm your stomach, despite being "weirdoughs and impastas"!

SAD KETO FLATBREAD $ ⚡ 🌿

If you are desperate for bread, especially at the start of your DIRTY, LAZY, KETO journey, give Sad Keto Flatbread a try. It's hard to transition away from breads and crackers; I understand! You need a grace period, right? Transition recipes like these can help fill the void. For me, I really had to back away from bread and cracker recipes altogether. Overall, I found eating "bread substitutes" triggered my desperate desire for Cheez-Its. I understand that not everyone is as addicted to snack foods as I am, so I'm sharing this Sad Keto Flatbread recipe for your consideration. Its name was inspired from mourning the loss of bread.

4 tablespoons coconut flour

2 tablespoons unblanched almond flour

4 tablespoons vital wheat gluten

½ teaspoon baking powder

⅛ teaspoon baking soda

¼ teaspoon salt

2 teaspoons grated Parmesan cheese

⅓ cup full-fat sour cream

1 Preheat oven to 450°F. Line a baking sheet with parchment paper.

2 In a small bowl, combine the flours, wheat gluten, baking powder, baking soda, salt, and Parmesan.

3 Add sour cream and stir thoroughly until dough forms. If your dough will not form, try adding a sprinkle of water.

4 Split mixture into two balls and place on baking sheet.

5 Cover dough with another piece of parchment paper and roll dough out to desired thickness (planning for it to rise slightly). Note that thinner dough will be crispier. Remove the top piece of parchment paper.

6 Bake 10 minutes (or longer for crispier texture), flipping after 5 minutes.

7 Remove from oven and serve warm.

NET CARBS
5G

SERVES 4

PER SERVING:

CALORIES	143
FAT	6G
PROTEIN	14G
SODIUM	282MG
FIBER	3G
CARBOHYDRATES	8G
SUGAR	2G

TIME

PREP TIME:	10 MIN
COOK TIME:	10 MIN

TIPS & OPTIONS

For added zing, brush your Sad Keto Flatbread with olive oil and sprinkle with lemon salt.

Make Sad Keto Flatbread a dessert by brushing the final product with melted butter, a sprinkle of cinnamon, and Splenda (or your favorite sugar substitute).

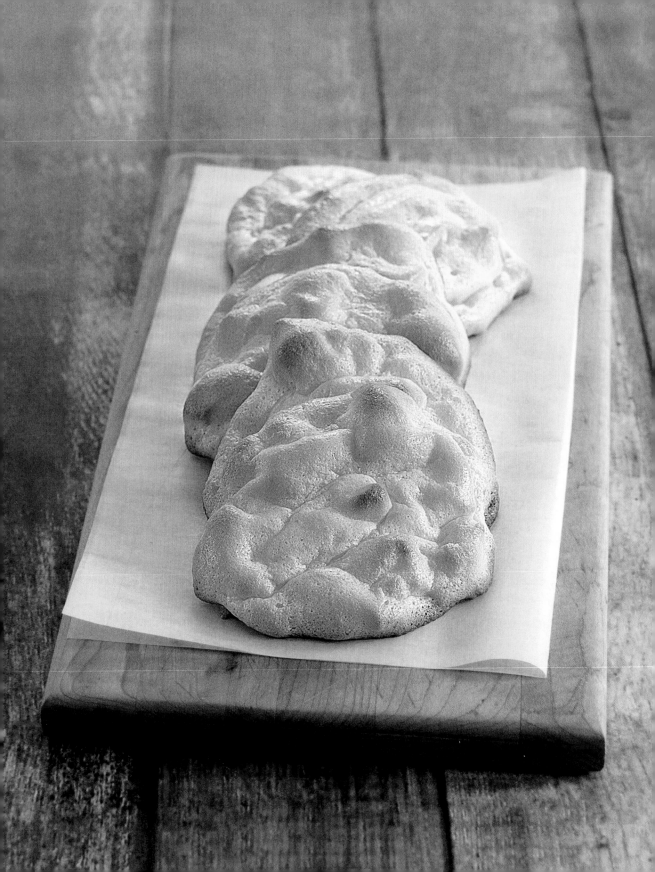

CONSOLATION PRIZE CLOUD BREAD

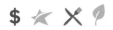

Cloud bread is one of the most talked about keto recipes (behind Fathead Pizza Crust, of course). Every keto beginner yearns for their beloved bread at first and is willing to spend time in the kitchen trying to magically create a low-carb version. I want to fore-warn you at this fork in the road (get it, fork?) that keto bread reci-pes will never taste like real bread. They aren't bad tasting, but they do taste different and have a unique texture. In order to not feel disappointed, I recommend you lower (or change) your expectations about keto bread substitutes.

3 tablespoons full-fat cream cheese, softened

3 large eggs

1 tablespoon 0g net carb sweetener

¼ teaspoon baking powder

1 Preheat oven to 300°F. Line a baking sheet with parchment paper.

2 In a medium microwave-safe bowl, microwave cream cheese 30 seconds. Stir and microwave again for 15 seconds.

3 Crack eggs and separate into two different medium bowls. Add cream cheese to the bowl containing the yolks, and add 0g net carb sweetener to the egg whites.

4 Combine baking powder with egg whites and beat with electric mixer until stiff peaks form, about 3–4 minutes at high speed. Make sure there is no yolk in bowl, as it will not mix properly.

5 Blend egg yolk mixture with a whisk or hand mixer until well blended and smooth. Cream cheese must be completely mixed in.

6 Gently fold egg yolk mixture into egg white mixture until fully combined.

7 Spoon mixture into six even patties on baking sheet. Bake 30–35 minutes until tops are golden.

8 Let cool 10 minutes and lift off parchment paper (easiest to do when rolls are still warm). Serve.

NET CARBS

1G

SERVES 6

PER SERVING:

CALORIES	60
FAT	4G
PROTEIN	4G
SODIUM	82MG
FIBER	0G
CARBOHYDRATES	1G
SUGAR	0G

TIME

PREP TIME:	10 MIN
COOK TIME:	36 MIN

TIPS & OPTIONS

Sprinkle with cheese, salt, and garlic.

These tasty buns can be served warm or cold.

Store in an airtight con-tainer or resealable bag. They last up to three days at room temperature and seven days in the fridge.

OG BREADSTICKS $

TIPS & OPTIONS

Sometimes the process of microwaving the cauliflower causes it to release water, making the mixture watery when blended. Dry out the blended cauliflower by patting the mixture with paper towels, squeezing inside of a cheesecloth, or draining in a colander.

A good rule to follow is to proceed only when the cauliflower mixture is solid enough to roll onto parchment paper. The oven will help with the rest of the drying.

*Cauliflower continues to amaze me. Along with the infamous avocado, **it's a keto superstar!** I love its simplicity, versatility, and ability to fill me up. Since I'm a volume eater, I include as many vegetables as I can into my diet to "slow down" my eating.*

4 cups riced cauliflower

2 cups shredded whole milk mozzarella cheese, divided

2 large eggs, whisked

1 tablespoon garlic powder

1 tablespoon Italian seasoning

1 Preheat oven to 450°F. Line a baking sheet with parchment paper.

2 In a medium microwave-safe bowl, microwave cauliflower 3–4 minutes to soften. Put in colander and let cool 5 minutes.

3 Add cauliflower to a food processor and pulse until consistency becomes a gritty pulp. Remove excess water by squeezing in a cheesecloth.

4 Pour cauliflower into a medium mixing bowl and add the rest of ingredients, leaving out ¼ cup of cheese to add at the end. Thoroughly mix ingredients in the bowl until they form a big ball of dough.

5 Place dough on baking sheet and top with another sheet of parchment paper.

6 Roll out dough until it's about ¼" thick. The shape doesn't matter. Don't worry if it's a little watery; the oven will firm it up.

7 Remove top piece of parchment paper and bake 20 minutes until it shows signs of browning.

8 Remove and top with remaining cheese. Cut with a pizza cutter and serve warm.

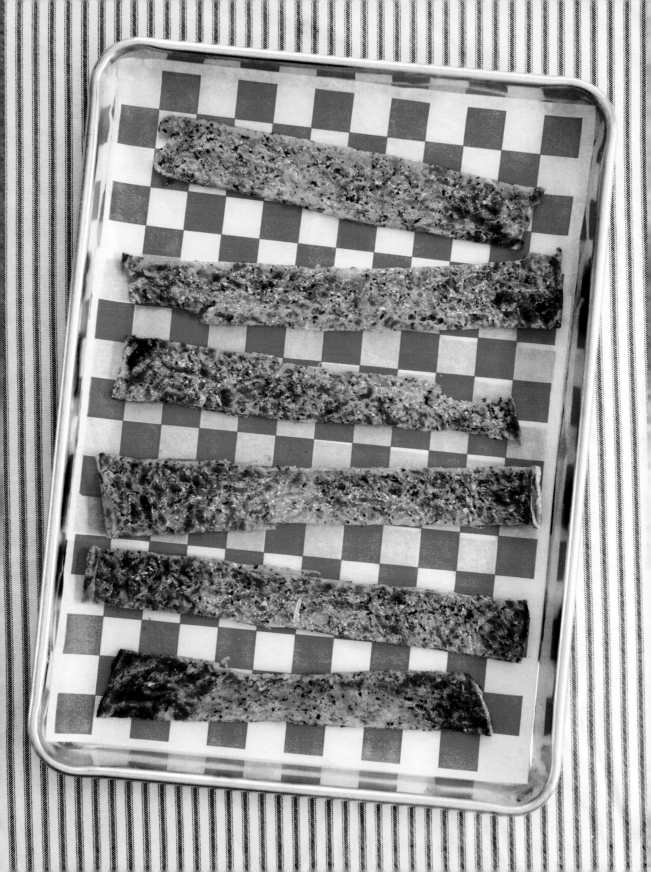

PIZZA HUT CHEESY BREADSTICKS $

Pizza Hut Cheesy Breadsticks are a variation of keto flatbread. If you are desperate for a bread fix, give this one a try!

2 cups shredded whole milk mozzarella, divided

1 ounce full-fat cream cheese, softened

½ cup blanched almond flour

3 tablespoons coconut flour

1 large egg, whisked

⅓ cup grated Parmesan cheese

1 teaspoon dried parsley

1 Preheat oven to 425°F.

2 In a large microwave-safe bowl, place 1½ cups mozzarella and cream cheese. Heat in microwave for 1½ minutes, stirring every 30 seconds.

3 Add almond flour, coconut flour, and egg. Fold until blended.

4 Let dough cool for handling. Form dough into a ball and place between two sheets of parchment paper. Roll out to approximately ¼" thick.

5 Remove top sheet of paper and place dough, while still on the bottom piece of parchment paper, on a baking sheet. Sprinkle ¼ cup mozzarella over dough. Bake 5–7 minutes until the edges of dough are golden.

6 Take dough out of oven. Sprinkle with remaining mozzarella and Parmesan cheese. Bake 5 minutes until cheese is melted.

7 Remove from oven and garnish with parsley. Cut into twelve equal breadsticks using a pizza cutter. Serve warm.

SEXY FETTUCCINI ALFREDO

*If you ever feel like you are somehow "missing out" while on your weight loss journey, pull out this recipe. You **can't possibly feel deprived** while eating the most delicious sauce on the planet. This Sexy Fettuccini Alfredo sauce is so heavenly and rich, you are sure to feel scandalous and downright sexy while eating it over your keto noodles.*

Keto Noodles

3 cups fine unblanched almond flour

⅓ cup coconut flour

6 teaspoons xanthan gum

6 teaspoons apple cider vinegar

3 large eggs, whisked

1 tablespoon water, if needed for consistency

Alfredo Sauce

½ cup unsalted butter

2 cloves garlic, peeled and minced

4 ounces full-fat cream cheese, softened

1½ cups heavy whipping cream

1½ cups grated Parmesan cheese

¼ teaspoon salt

NET CARBS	
9G	

SERVES 8	

PER SERVING:	
CALORIES	701
FAT	60G
PROTEIN	20G
SODIUM	526MG
FIBER	9G
CARBOHYDRATES	18G
SUGAR	4G

TIME	
PREP TIME:	50 MIN
COOK TIME:	28 MIN

1   Preheat oven to 375°F. Line a baking sheet with parchment paper.

2   In a large mixing bowl, mix dry noodle ingredients together. Add vinegar and eggs and mix thoroughly. If the dough is too thick, add a bit of water (very slowly) to reach desired consistency.

3   Refrigerate dough 30 minutes.

4   Put the chilled dough ball in center of the baking sheet and cover dough with second piece of parchment paper. Using rolling pin, roll to desired noodle thickness.

5   Remove top piece of parchment paper. Using a pizza cutter, cut dough into thin strips for noodles. Bake 20 minutes until noodles are firm, but loose, like pasta.

6   Make the sauce: Melt butter in a medium saucepan over medium heat. Add garlic and cook 3 minutes until soft. Add remaining sauce ingredients while stirring until cheese is completely melted and a thick, uniform sauce forms (about 5 minutes).

7   Top each keto noodle serving with ½ cup Alfredo sauce. Serve.

TIPS & OPTIONS

Instead of making noodles from scratch, substitute "zoodles," or zucchini noodles. Whether you purchase zoodles or make them from scratch, the trick to al dente cooking is to lightly sauté the zoodles with a tablespoon of oil in a frying pan (as opposed to steaming them, which causes them to become mushy). Zoodles will greatly reduce your net carbs per serving when compared to pasta.

For added protein, toss cubed cooked chicken into your Alfredo sauce.

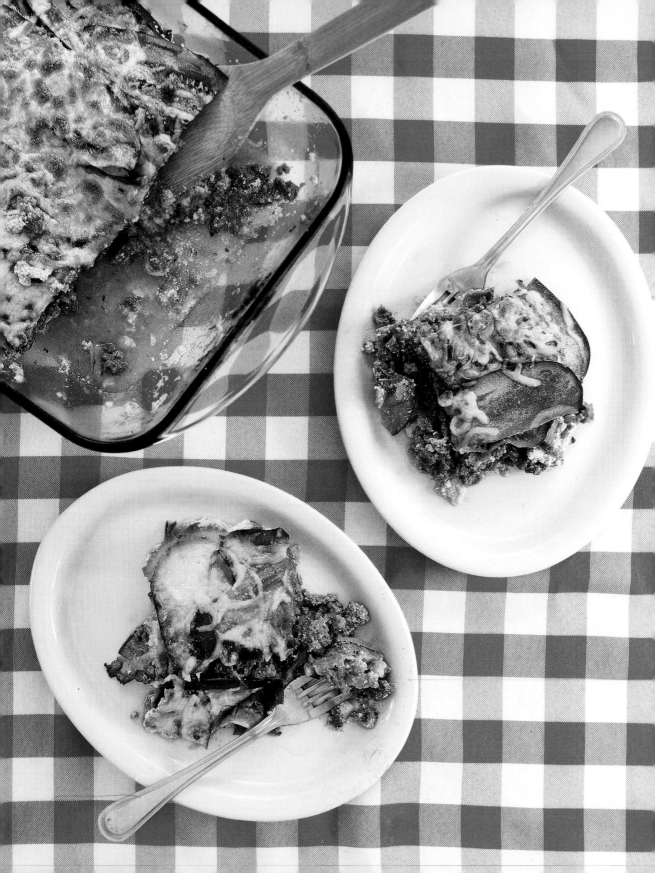

PURPLE EGGPLANT LASAGNA

This comforting, hearty dish is best enjoyed during the winter months. A casserole-style meal like this warms the soul as well as your home while it's cooking. When I'm feeling blue or a little down because it's cold outside, Purple Eggplant Lasagna fills a culinary hole in my heart. Food might not equal love, but sometimes its warmth hits the right spot.

1 pound lean ground beef

½ medium onion, peeled and chopped

¼ cup dried parsley

1 cup no-sugar-added pasta sauce

1 pound whole milk ricotta cheese

1 large egg, whisked

⅛ teaspoon salt

⅛ teaspoon black pepper

1 large eggplant

2 cups shredded whole milk mozzarella cheese, divided

1. Preheat oven to 350°F. Grease a 13" × 9" casserole dish.

2. In a large skillet over medium heat, brown beef 10–15 minutes until cooked thoroughly. Drain fat. Add onion and parsley and cook 2–3 minutes until soft. Add pasta sauce and bring to boil while stirring frequently (3–5 minutes). Turn off heat.

3. In a medium bowl, mix ricotta cheese and egg and then season with salt and pepper.

4. Cut unpeeled eggplant lengthwise in thin slices no more than ⅛". You should have enough for two complete layers in your baking dish.

5. In the casserole dish, add ¼" layer of ricotta cheese mixture to prevent eggplant from sticking. On top of ricotta layer, make an even layer of half the eggplant slices.

6. Spread a layer of half of the remaining ricotta cheese mixture.

7. Next, spread 1 cup mozzarella cheese, then half of the meat/pasta sauce and the rest of the eggplant, followed by the rest of the ricotta mixture and leftover meat mixture. Finally, top with remaining 1 cup mozzarella cheese.

8. Cover dish with foil. Bake 40 minutes. Remove the foil and cook an additional 5 minutes to brown cheese.

9. Let cool 15 minutes, then cut and serve.

NET CARBS

5G

SERVES 10

PER SERVING:

CALORIES	250
FAT	14G
PROTEIN	21G
SODIUM	381MG
FIBER	3G
CARBOHYDRATES	8G
SUGAR	3G

TIME

PREP TIME:	30 MIN
COOK TIME:	68 MIN

TIPS & OPTIONS

Eggplant skin will soften as it cooks.

Microwave the thinly sliced eggplant prior to making the lasagna (about 3–4 minutes) to prevent your final product from tasting "woody."

Add cooked Italian sausage to your sauce to increase protein.

Vegetable lasagna tends to become a bit more "watery" than traditional noodle lasagna. Rest assured, the excess liquid dissipates with subsequent reheating.

Make this dish vegetarian by omitting meat or substituting tofu for beef.

HOMETOWN BUFFET MAC-N-CHEESE $

NET CARBS

6G

SERVES 4

PER SERVING:

CALORIES	397
FAT	33G
PROTEIN	14G
SODIUM	750MG
FIBER	2G
CARBOHYDRATES	8G
SUGAR	4G

TIME

PREP TIME:	20 MIN
COOK TIME:	37 MIN

TIPS & OPTIONS ≫

If you are in a hurry (who isn't?), then don't steam the cauliflower on the stovetop. Microwave the cauliflower in a large microwave-safe glass dish with ½ cup water for 4–6 minutes until it is the desired softness.

This recipe isn't just for the kids in your household. Spice up your serving with a sprinkle of cayenne pepper to add color and kick.

For added presentation drama, sometimes I make this dish in a cast iron pan. After creating the recipe, I put the entire pan into my oven with the broiler on high to brown the cheese until crispy.

*Because I eat large portions, I have to watch myself around cheesy dishes. Even though I count only net carbs, I'm still conscious of the caloric damage dairy products can wreak on my waistline! Instead of eating cheese for cheese's sake, I enjoy it **as a topping** on vegetables. Cheese, a delicious fat, makes every vegetable taste **like a rock star**. Even my kids, the pickiest of eaters, enjoy my version of Hometown Buffet Mac-n-Cheese.*

1 pound cauliflower, chopped into small florets

1 cup grated low-fat Parmesan cheese

½ cup heavy whipping cream

¾ cup shredded Cheddar cheese

2 ounces full-fat cream cheese, cubed

2 tablespoons olive oil

2 teaspoons Dijon mustard

½ teaspoon garlic powder

⅛ teaspoon salt

⅛ teaspoon black pepper

1 Preheat oven to 400°F. Grease a 9" × 9" baking dish.

2 In a medium covered pot over medium heat, steam cauliflower 10–15 minutes or until softened to desired level.

3 Mix remaining ingredients in a large saucepan over medium heat and heat 5–7 minutes while stirring until cheeses are fully melted and blended.

4 Gently fold in steamed cauliflower, careful to maintain the shape of florets until fully coated.

5 Pour mixture into baking dish and bake 15 minutes (or until cheese turns golden brown).

6 Let cool 10 minutes and cut into serving sizes. Your dish is ready to serve.

LEGENDARY FATHEAD PIZZA CRUST

$ ★ ✕ ✿

And now we have for you, ladies and gentlemen, the world-famous (albeit only in the keto world,) Fathead Pizza Crust! This is probably one of the simplest recipes of the cookbook with very few ingredients and a prep time of only fifteen minutes. This recipe could become your most revisited page of the entire book!

1 cup unblanched almond flour

2 cups shredded whole milk mozzarella cheese

2 tablespoons full-fat cream cheese, softened

1 large egg

¼ teaspoon salt

1 Preheat oven to 425°F.

2 In a large microwave-safe bowl, combine almond flour with mozzarella cheese. Add softened cream cheese and microwave for 1 minute. Stir and microwave 30 seconds.

3 Thoroughly mix in egg and salt.

4 Remove dough from bowl and form into ball with your hands. Place dough between two large pieces of parchment paper. Roll dough into circular crust, about ¼" in thickness.

5 Remove the top piece of parchment paper and place the formed crust with parchment paper under it on a baking pan.

6 Bake 10–14 minutes until top starts to turn brown.

NET CARBS

2G

SERVES 8	
PER SERVING:	
CALORIES	185
FAT	14G
PROTEIN	10G
SODIUM	270MG
FIBER	2G
CARBOHYDRATES	4G
SUGAR	1G

TIME	
PREP TIME:	15 MIN
COOK TIME:	16 MIN

TIPS & OPTIONS

For a crispier crust, omit the egg.

As bubbles form during baking, pop with a fork.

Suggestions for sauce: no-sugar-added marinara sauce, homemade keto-friendly pizza sauce, pesto, or Alfredo sauce.

Dice up broccoli, zucchini, spinach, mushrooms, and black olives to create a "veggie lovers"–style pizza.

LITTLE ITALY BAKED ZITI

*I used to think Italian food was "off limits" on DIRTY, LAZY, KETO until I created this recipe. The trick for making Little Italy Baked Ziti is to **not overcook** the cauliflower. The florets need to be firm enough to hold up when folding with the other ingredients, or else they turn mushy. Little Italy Baked Ziti is great for leftovers since the casserole is easy to reheat. The presentation looks almost like a cheese lasagna, so be prepared to share with even the pickiest eaters in your household.*

1 pound Italian sausage links, diced

1 tablespoon olive oil

1 small white onion, peeled and chopped

2 cloves garlic, peeled and minced

¼ teaspoon salt

⅛ teaspoon black pepper

1 (24-ounce) can no-sugar-added pasta sauce

2 medium heads cauliflower, cut into florets

2 cups whole milk ricotta cheese

2 cups shredded whole milk mozzarella cheese

½ cup grated low-fat Parmesan cheese

1　Preheat oven to 350°F. Grease a 9" × 13" glass pan.

2　In a medium skillet over medium heat, sauté Italian sausage with oil, onion, garlic, salt, and pepper. Cook until browned. Do not drain fat.

3　Stir in pasta sauce and cook 2 more minutes. Reduce heat to medium-low and simmer 10 minutes with lid on.

4　In a medium pot over a medium heat, lightly steam cauliflower florets 10–15 minutes until they soften and hold their shape and do not become mushy.

5　In a large mixing bowl, gently fold cauliflower with meat sauce.

6　Pour half of the mixture into glass pan and sprinkle with half of the three cheeses.

7　Spread remaining cauliflower mix in the glass pan and top with the remaining half of the three cheeses.

8　Bake 30 minutes. Cool and serve.

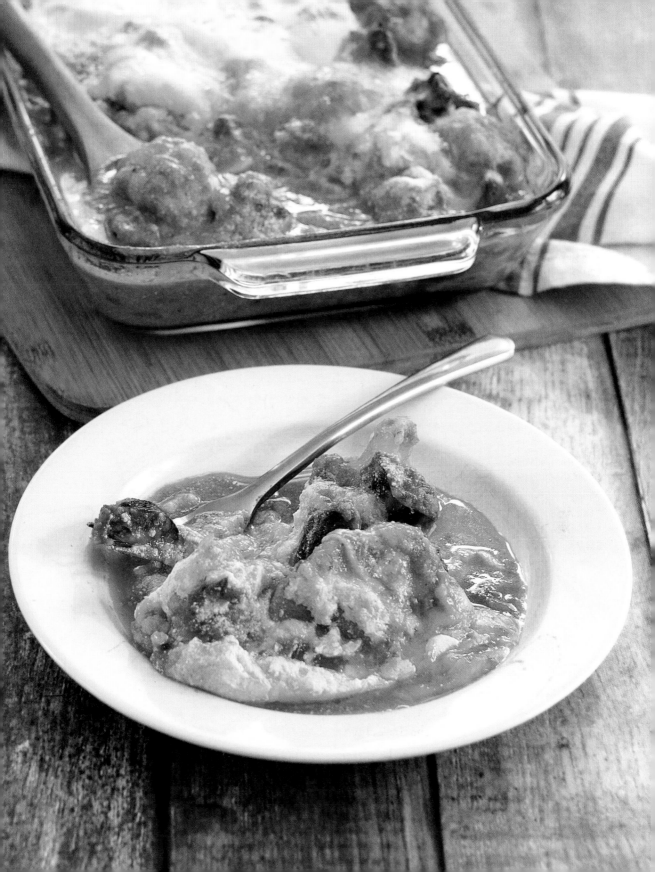

INSTANT PROTEIN PIZZA CRUST

$

NET CARBS

2G

SERVES 6

PER SERVING:

CALORIES	148
FAT	7G
PROTEIN	16G
SODIUM	419MG
FIBER	0G
CARBOHYDRATES	2G
SUGAR	0G

TIME

PREP TIME:	5 MIN
COOK TIME:	20 MIN

TIPS & OPTIONS

Suggestions for sauce: no-sugar-added marinara sauce, homemade keto-friendly pizza sauce, pesto, or Alfredo sauce.

Dice up broccoli, zucchini, spinach, mushrooms, and black olives to create a "veggie lovers"–style pizza.

You can use your hands (or press the dough with the bottom of a skillet) if you don't have a rolling pin. The pizza crust will be covered with toppings anyway; it doesn't have to look pretty.

As an alternate to the Legendary Fathead Pizza Crust (see recipe in this chapter), Instant Protein Pizza Crust offers variety and a powerful protein boost. This recipe got me excited because it was the first time in my life I turned my oven up to 500°F. THAT'S HOT STUFF!

1 (10-ounce) can chicken, drained
1 large egg
½ cup grated Parmesan cheese
¼ cup shredded whole milk mozzarella cheese

1　Preheat oven to 350°F.

2　Line a baking sheet with parchment paper and thinly spread chicken onto paper. Place in oven and heat 10 minutes to dry chicken.

3　Remove chicken from oven and scrape into a medium mixing bowl. Increase temperature of oven to 500°F.

4　Add egg, Parmesan cheese, and mozzarella cheese to chicken. Mix well to form a ball of dough.

5　Line a baking sheet again with parchment paper and place dough in middle. Cover with second sheet of parchment paper. Use a rolling pin to create a thin round crust.

6　Remove top piece of parchment paper and bake 8–10 minutes until crust browns. Be patient during this step to ensure a crispy pizza crust later!

7　Remove from the oven.

SLOW YOUR ROLL PIZZA CRUST $

*Because we all love pizza, it's important to try out multiple recipes in order to find the best "fit." Each DIRTY, LAZY, KETO pizza recipe is slightly different. In my experience, you must find something that works **for you**! Even though the Slow Your Roll Pizza Crust has more of a moist crust than the other recipes, I sleep better knowing I ate more vegetables using this recipe. Also, because I tend to overeat pizza, adding cauliflower as a main ingredient helps slow down my eating! This vegetarian crust helps me to eat fewer pizza slices overall, so it quickly became one of my favorites.*

3 cups riced cauliflower

1 large egg, beaten

½ teaspoon garlic powder

1½ cups shredded whole milk mozzarella, divided

¼ cup grated Parmesan cheese

½ teaspoon dried basil

½ teaspoon dried oregano

¼ teaspoon salt

1 cup no-sugar-added pasta sauce

NET CARBS
4G

SERVES 8	
PER SERVING:	
CALORIES	106
FAT	6G
PROTEIN	8G
SODIUM	357MG
FIBER	1G
CARBOHYDRATES	5G
SUGAR	3G

TIME	
PREP TIME:	20 MIN
COOK TIME:	24 MIN

1. Preheat oven to 500°F. Line a baking sheet with parchment paper.

2. In a medium microwave-safe bowl, microwave riced cauliflower 3–4 minutes. Remove from microwave and let cool 5–10 minutes.

3. Place cauliflower on a clean kitchen towel and squeeze out excess moisture.

4. In a medium bowl, combine cauliflower with beaten egg, garlic powder, 1 cup mozzarella cheese, Parmesan, basil, oregano, and salt. Stir and fold until dough forms.

5. Place dough ball on baking sheet. Use hands or rolling pin to flatten dough to ¼" flat circle.

6. Bake 10–15 minutes or until crust is golden and crispy.

7. Remove from oven. Add pasta sauce first and then remaining mozzarella cheese.

8. Return to oven 3–5 minutes to melt cheese.

TIPS & OPTIONS

I recommend utilizing every eating opportunity as a way to sneak in more vegetables. Just last night, I made this pizza with Alfredo sauce, but then topped it with half a bag of shredded broccoli mix. The resulting pizza looked like something I might order at California Pizza Kitchen. I impressed even myself!

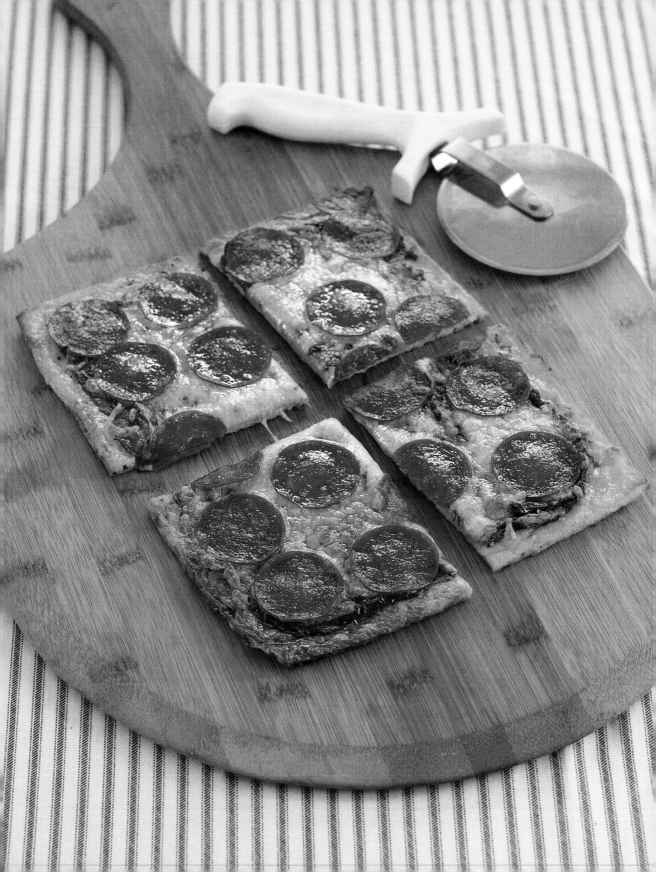

FAST TWO-STEP PIZZA $ ✕

Have you ever seen someone eat two pieces of pizza, one on top of the other, like a sandwich? I've always been irritated by that technique—who is in such a hurry that they need to double-team their slices? Perhaps I'm in awe. I wish my metabolism could handle that kind of eating. I work hard at consciously slowing down my chewing as I often finish my plate without any memories of actually eating! Enjoy your food slowly, but cook quickly. If you're in a hurry, or have run out of almond flour, the Fast Two-Step Pizza crust comes to the rescue. It's simple and fast, yet crispy and delicious!

Crust
4 large eggs

1½ cups shredded whole milk mozzarella cheese

Toppings
3 tablespoons tomato paste

1 teaspoon dried oregano

1¼ cups shredded whole milk mozzarella cheese

2 ounces sliced pepperoni

1 Preheat oven to 400°F. Line a baking sheet with parchment paper.

2 For the crust, mix eggs and 1½ cups of mozzarella cheese in a medium bowl. Stir thoroughly.

3 Spread egg batter on baking sheet, creating one large pizza crust or two smaller ones.

4 Bake 15 minutes until crust is golden and firm. Remove and let cool.

5 Raise the oven temperature to 450°F.

6 For the toppings, spread tomato paste on crust and sprinkle oregano on top. Top with even layer of mozzarella cheese and evenly distribute pepperoni.

7 Bake 5–10 minutes until cheese starts to turn golden.

8 Remove from oven and serve right away.

NET CARBS	
3G	

SERVES 6	
PER SERVING:	
CALORIES	255
FAT	17G
PROTEIN	18G
SODIUM	598MG
FIBER	0G
CARBOHYDRATES	3G
SUGAR	2G

TIME	
PREP TIME:	10 MIN
COOK TIME:	25 MIN

≪ TIPS & OPTIONS

Sneak more vegetables into your diet with creative low-carb toppings: spinach, broccoli, zucchini, or mushrooms.

Even though it's a DIRTY, LAZY, KETO recipe, pizza dishes are still *easy to overeat*. Adding vegetables to your meal, either as a topping or on the side, will help you to "slow your roll."

CHAPTER 7

SIDES

Slow your roll. One secret of adulthood I've learned along my weight loss journey is to *"eat ya vegetables."* Eating vegetables is like going to the dentist. Every time I make the decision to eat them, I feel responsible, like a real grown-up. I will even go so far as to admit feeling smug in line at the grocery store when I load vegetables onto the conveyer belt. I feel proud for investing in my health (*so obnoxious, I know!*). My core motivation for eating vegetables, though, is much more devious. The reason I eat so many vegetables is that they actually *slow down my eating.* I lack an internal "off switch" that tells me when I'm full. *I will eat, and eat, and eat, until physically, I can't eat any more.* Vegetables, by adding serious fiber to my meals, quickly swell in my stomach and stop the madness from continuing. The Sides recipes I've shared here in this cookbook capitalize on what vegetables do for the body. This is such a different approach to eating than how I grew up.

GREEN "POTATO" BOATS

NET CARBS

5G

SERVES 4

PER SERVING:

CALORIES	259
FAT	20G
PROTEIN	10G
SODIUM	496MG
FIBER	1G
CARBOHYDRATES	6G
SUGAR	4G

TIME

PREP TIME:	10 MIN
COOK TIME:	30 MIN

TIPS & OPTIONS

Choose wider zucchini to prevent breakage when scooping out the insides.

Don't overstuff your zucchini, or you won't have enough for the entire recipe.

Optional garnishes to consider: finely chopped green onion (the green part) or full-fat sour cream.

How to prep a jalapeño pepper: First, wash the pepper and cut off the stem. Cut lengthwise down the middle. With a spoon, scrape out the seeds and white tissue that is also on the inside (deveining). This process removes most of the heat from the pepper.

Twice-baked potatoes? I used to think cauliflower was the only substitute for mashed potatoes. Surprisingly, mashed zucchini makes an excellent alternative. As an added bonus, I've discovered that my kids will eat anything served to them in a boat! If this is your first time prepping a jalapeño for this recipe, be sure to wash your hands thoroughly to prevent "jalapeño hands," **which is a real thing**—*Google it!*

2 medium zucchini

½ cup grated Cheddar cheese

2 ounces full-fat cream cheese, softened

¼ cup diced onion

¼ cup full-fat sour cream

2 tablespoons melted unsalted butter

¼ teaspoon salt

4 strips no-sugar-added bacon, cooked and crumbled

1 medium jalapeño pepper, deveined, seeded, and finely chopped

1 Preheat oven to 350°F.

2 Cut the zucchini in half lengthwise. Cut in half again at the midpoint to create eight "boats" 3"–4" long to be hollowed out.

3 With a spoon, scoop out each boat; try to get most out but leave enough so the sides aren't too thin (about ¼" max). Chop the removed flesh finely and put in a medium bowl.

4 Place eight scooped-out boats in a large greased baking dish.

5 Add remaining ingredients except bacon and jalapeños to bowl with zucchini flesh and mix well. Divide mixture evenly and scoop into the boats.

6 Top with crumbled bacon and jalapeño.

7 Bake 30 minutes until filling bubbles and zucchini boats are softened.

8 Remove from oven and let cool 5 minutes. Serve.

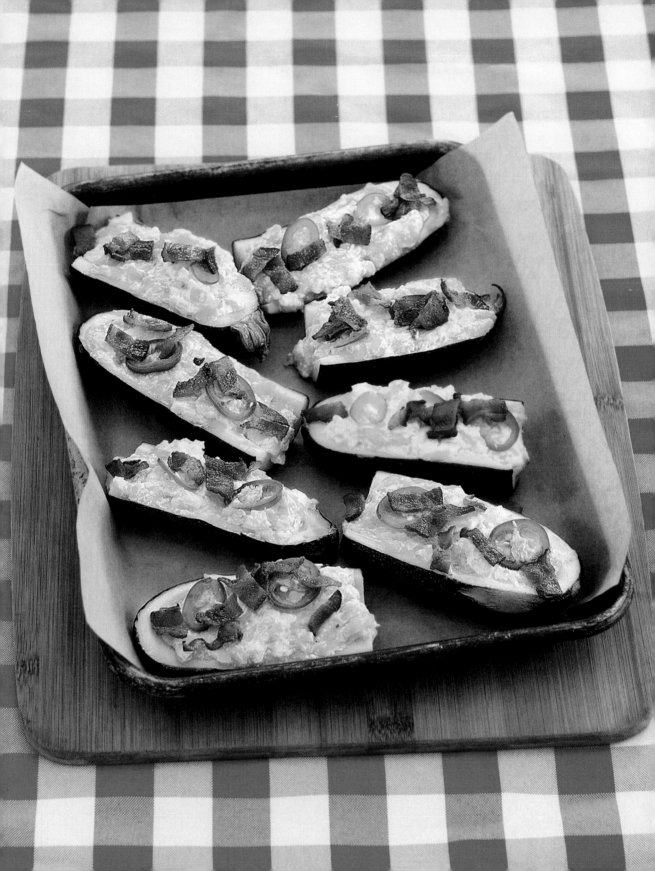

ACADEMY PARMESAN CAULIFLOWER

$ ✕ 🌱

TIPS & OPTIONS

In a hurry? Decrease the required cook time by microwaving raw cauliflower for a few minutes prior to starting the recipe. This will soften the cauliflower and speed up overall cook time.

For all the spicy food lovers, try coating roasted cauliflower with Buffalo hot sauce or Cajun spices and enjoy while watching the game.

Be creative with your cauliflower toppings. One of my favorites is to toss roasted cauliflower with store-bought pesto sauce.

"And the Academy Award goes to…" CAULIFLOWER! *In my opinion, cauliflower beats the avocado for being the poster child for DIRTY, LAZY, KETO. It's an inexpensive, versatile vegetable that can take on the flavor of a dish it's part of, or stand tall on its own. Whether served raw, mashed, roasted, or riced, cauliflower stole my heart years ago.*

16 ounces cauliflower, cut into bite-sized florets

4 tablespoons melted unsalted butter

2 tablespoons olive oil

¼ teaspoon salt

¼ teaspoon black pepper

1 cup grated Parmesan cheese

2 teaspoons parsley flakes

1. Preheat oven to 400°F. Line a baking sheet with parchment paper.

2. In a large mixing bowl, toss cauliflower, melted butter, and olive oil. Add salt and pepper.

3. Place coated cauliflower on the baking sheet. Keep cauliflower in a single layer so it cooks evenly. Bake 25–30 minutes or until soft.

4. Remove from oven and dust with Parmesan cheese and parsley. Return to oven for 5 minutes to melt cheese.

5. Remove from the oven and serve warm.

DUCAT PESTO PASTA

*When basil is in season, I buy pillows of fresh leaves at every produce stand for **a ducat**! (My teenage daughter taught me that slang word, which means "a dollar.") Making pesto from scratch is super easy, though only affordable (in my opinion) when the leaves are in season. Otherwise, I encourage you to buy a premade jar of pesto at your local big-box store or supermarket. It's worth the investment to always have a jar in your fridge.*

¼ cup pine nuts

4 cloves garlic, peeled and chopped

1½ cups fresh basil leaves

½ cup olive oil

½ cup grated or shredded Parmesan cheese, divided

1 large head cauliflower, cut into bite-sized florets

1   Pulse the pine nuts, garlic, basil, oil, and ¼ cup Parmesan cheese in a small blender until liquefied, about 1–2 minutes.

2   Steam cauliflower florets until tender, about 10–15 minutes.

3   Place florets in a medium mixing bowl and gently fold in pesto sauce.

4   Serve warm and sprinkle with remaining Parmesan cheese.

NET CARBS

7G

SERVES 6

PER SERVING:

CALORIES	270
FAT	23G
PROTEIN	6G
SODIUM	193MG
FIBER	3G
CARBOHYDRATES	10G
SUGAR	3G

TIME

PREP TIME:	5 MIN
COOK TIME:	15 MIN

TIPS & OPTIONS

To speed up the cooking process, microwave cauliflower for 4 minutes *and then* add the pesto, skipping the steaming. Make sure you like the softness of the cauliflower before adding the sauce.

This sauce freezes well. I freeze extra sauce using an ice cube tray. The cubes can then be easily added to future recipes.

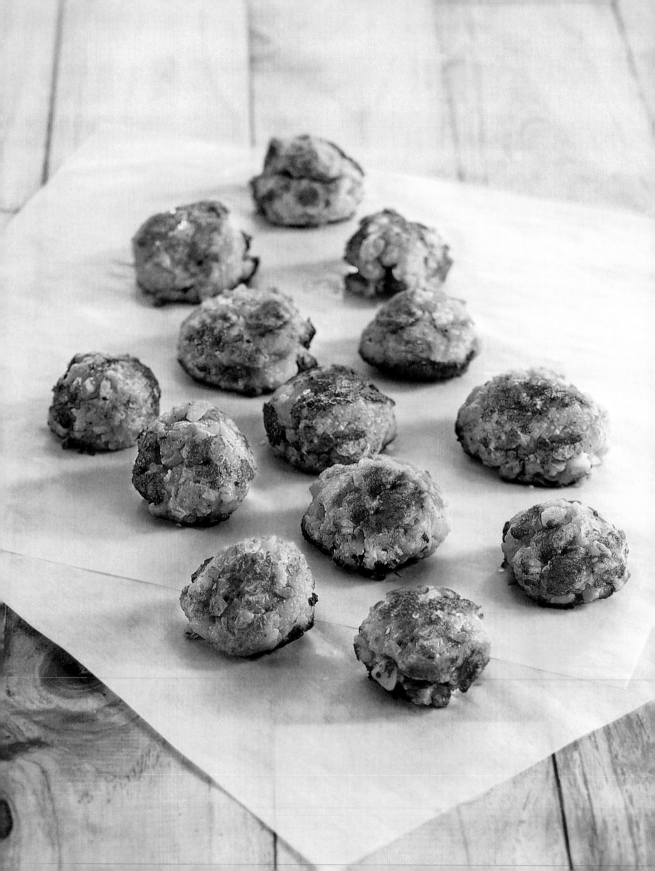

CAULIFLOWER TATER TOTS $ ✕ 🌿

Frozen Tater Tots and breaded Tyson chicken breasts were a staple of my teenage years. When I rebelled against the family dinner, I turned to either a bowl of cereal or frozen dinner made in the toaster oven (the era before the microwave!). Tater Tots feel like the redneck cousin of the French fry. Oh, how I love that pop of grease and salt! These Cauliflower Tater Tots come pretty close to the real thing, if you don't mind the prep work.

1½ pounds riced cauliflower

4 tablespoons avocado oil, divided

1 large egg

1½ cups shredded whole milk mozzarella

2 cloves minced garlic

¾ teaspoon salt, divided

1 In a large skillet over medium heat, fry cauliflower rice with 2 tablespoons oil for 5–10 minutes until soft and starting to brown. Turn off heat.

2 In a large bowl, whisk egg and mix in cheese, garlic, and ½ teaspoon salt.

3 Combine browned cauliflower rice with egg mixture. Stir mixture well to melt cheese. Form tots using a spoon or melon scoop.

4 In a large skillet over medium heat, fry tots using remaining 2 tablespoons oil. Space tots apart in a single layer, turning every 3–5 minutes, until browned on all sides.

5 Repeat until all tots are cooked. Sprinkle with remaining ¼ teaspoon salt and serve hot.

NET CARBS	
3G	
SERVES 8	
PER SERVING:	
CALORIES	154
FAT	12G
PROTEIN	7G
SODIUM	378MG
FIBER	2G
CARBOHYDRATES	5G
SUGAR	2G

TIME	
PREP TIME:	5 MIN
COOK TIME:	30 MIN

TIPS & OPTIONS

Enjoy Cauliflower Tater Tots with a dip in no-sugar-added ketchup, sugar-free barbecue sauce, or ranch dressing.

Feel extra "dirty"? Enjoy a bunless hot dog with your Cauliflower Tater Tots.

Make this dish more "grown-up" by topping it with sour cream, cheese, bacon, and even jalapeños.

BILL'S FRIED ZUCK PATTIES $

TIPS & OPTIONS ≫

The secret to making delicious fried zuck patties is patience. You must allow time for the mixture to properly drain. Let the mixture sit in a large colander for as long as you can stand it before getting to work. Getting rid of excess liquid helps the fried patties stick together during the cooking process.

Eggs and cheese are the "glue" that holds these patties together when frying. If you don't like the way the first couple patties hold together, add more cheese or an additional egg to the rest of the mixture.

Shredding zucchini by hand is no joke! If you happen to have a kitchen tool that efficiently shreds zucchini, now is the time to get it out of the box. This recipe can be time-consuming. I have been known to become impatient after making dozens of these patties. I've even gone to such extreme measures as to dump all the remaining mixture into the pan at once, creating a final, mega "zuck" cake! As long as the patty is thin, this method is still effective.

1 pound zucchini

1 teaspoon salt

2 large beaten eggs

2 medium green onions, chopped

1½ teaspoons lemon pepper

1 cup shredded whole milk mozzarella cheese

½ cup blanched almond flour

¼ cup grated Parmesan cheese

¼ cup flaxseed meal

4 tablespoons coconut oil

1 Grate zucchini and sprinkle with salt. Drain grated zucchini 15 minutes or more in a large colander. Turn shreds often to speed up drainage. Squeeze mixture using a cheesecloth to remove excess moisture.

2 In a large bowl, mix grated zucchini with beaten eggs and green onions.

3 In a small bowl, combine remaining ingredients except the oil. Add to zucchini mixture, stirring well.

4 Form "zuck" patties that are 3" in diameter and ½" thick.

5 In a large pan over medium heat, heat oil. Fry patties 3–5 minutes per side (this may take several flips).

6 When "zuck" patties are thoroughly cooked and firm throughout, place on a paper towel–lined plate to drain and cool.

ZUCCHINI FRENCH FRIES $ ✕ 🌿

*The desire to eat French fries haunts us all. Rather than licking the bottom of a McDonald's bag (**which I have done**), I suggest a zucchini spear alternative. Sure, you can grill zucchini on the barbecue, but when you're in the mood for something more rebellious, give this recipe a whirl!*

2 medium zucchini

¼ teaspoon salt

¼ teaspoon black pepper

¼ teaspoon garlic powder

¾ cup grated Parmesan cheese

1 large egg, beaten

1 Preheat oven to 425°F. Line a baking sheet with foil. Place a rack onto baking sheet to keep zucchini crispy.

2 Keep slicing each zucchini in half, lengthwise, until you have created eight long sticks of similar size. Then cut sticks in half again across the middle, making sixteen pieces (per zucchini).

3 In a medium bowl, mix salt, pepper, garlic powder, and cheese together. In a separate medium bowl add the beaten egg. First, dip each stick in the egg (shaking off excess). Second, press each side into the spices.

4 Place spaced apart on the rack in a single layer.

5 Bake 20 minutes, flipping fries and rotating pan halfway through until browned and crispy.

6 Turn oven to broil and broil 2–3 minutes until dark golden.

NET CARBS	
5G	

SERVES 4	
PER SERVING:	
CALORIES	113
FAT	6G
PROTEIN	8G
SODIUM	509MG
FIBER	1G
CARBOHYDRATES	6G
SUGAR	3G

TIME	
PREP TIME:	10 MIN
COOK TIME:	23 MIN

TIPS & OPTIONS

Ranch dressing for dipping is a must!

RADISH POTATOES IN DRAG

TIPS & OPTIONS

Sour cream is a great topping for your baked radishes.

If you prefer a crispier texture, give this suggestion a try. Toss your cooked radishes with olive oil and place under the broiler until golden brown, turning every few minutes to crisp every side.

*It was years, YEARS, before I discovered the secret benefit of radishes; yes, you heard me right—I said **RADISHES**! It's almost unbelievable how similar to a boiled potato a radish can look **and taste** after it's been well cooked. RADISHES! How weird is that? As an added bonus, raw radishes are inexpensive and seem to last forever in the fridge.*

20 medium radishes, trimmed and halved

2 tablespoons olive oil

2 teaspoons Italian seasoning, divided

¼ teaspoon salt

¼ teaspoon black pepper

¼ cup grated Parmesan cheese

1 Preheat oven to 400°F. Grease a large baking dish with olive oil.

2 Add halved radishes to baking dish, brush with olive oil, and dust with half of the Italian seasoning, salt, and pepper.

3 Bake 45 minutes until light brown and crisp. Toss and re-season halfway through.

4 Add Parmesan on top and bake 5 more minutes. Remove from the oven and your golden radishes are ready to serve.

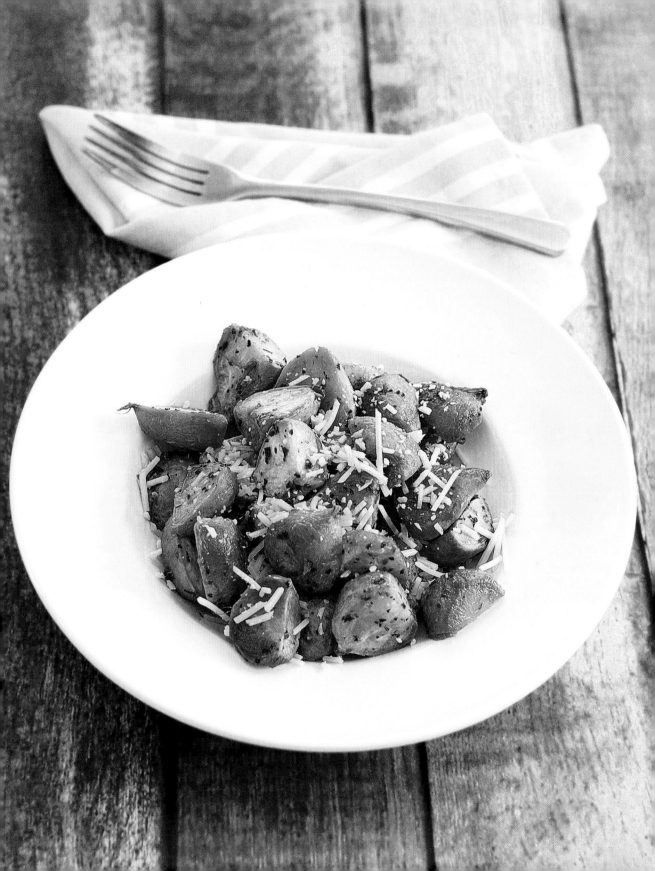

GET LOADED SMASHED CAULIFLOWER

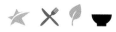

TIPS & OPTIONS

Bacon can be added to the top for better flavor and appearance.

Top with gravy? No one will ever recognize these mashed potatoes in disguise.

When cauliflower is on sale, I make this recipe in bulk and freeze inside large Ziploc bags.

In lieu of chopped green onion, you can substitute ranch powder.

Get Loaded Smashed Cauliflower is my favorite side dish! The varieties are endless. I change the recipe often according to the ingredients I have on hand, and have never been disappointed. For example, I have used these "fats" interchangeably: sour cream, half and half, cream cheese, butter, or heavy whipping cream.

1 pound cauliflower florets

3 tablespoons unsalted butter

¼ teaspoon garlic powder

½ cup fat-free sour cream

2 tablespoons chopped green onion, divided

1 cup shredded Cheddar cheese, divided

¼ teaspoon salt

1. Steam florets 10–15 minutes until very soft. Remove from heat and let sit in metal colander for 10–15 minutes to release water.

2. Pulse florets in a food processor 2–3 minutes until fluffy. Add butter, garlic powder, and sour cream and process 2–3 more minutes until it resembles mashed potatoes.

3. Scoop cauliflower into a medium microwave-safe bowl and mix in two-thirds of the green onion and ½ cup cheese and salt. Microwave 2–3 minutes.

4. Serve and sprinkle remaining cheese and green onion on top.

GRANDMA-MAH'S CREAMED SPINACH

   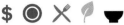

*One of the reasons I have been so successful with DIRTY, LAZY, KETO is that it doesn't feel "like a diet." The foods are **rich, luxurious, and decadent**. To outsiders, DIRTY, LAZY, KETO dishes don't appear to be "diet food." Creamed spinach is a perfect example! Whether it's served on a special holiday or alongside a family meal, I enjoy Grandma-Mah's Creamed Spinach often without any guilt.*

20 ounces fresh spinach, finely chopped

⅓ cup grated Parmesan cheese

6 ounces full-fat cream cheese, softened

4 tablespoons full-fat sour cream

½ teaspoon garlic powder

½ teaspoon onion powder

¼ teaspoon salt

¼ teaspoon black pepper

1 In a large nonstick saucepan over medium heat, add spinach. Cook 3–5 minutes while stirring until wilted and excess water is removed.

2 Add remaining ingredients and stir 5–10 minutes until cheeses are melted and ingredients are blended. Serve.

NET CARBS
4G

SERVES 6

PER SERVING:

CALORIES	158
FAT	11G
PROTEIN	6G
SODIUM	378MG
FIBER	2G
CARBOHYDRATES	6G
SUGAR	2G

TIME

PREP TIME:	5 MIN
COOK TIME:	15 MIN

TIPS & OPTIONS

Save time and buy pre-washed, precut spinach.

CHAPTER 8

MAIN DISHES

Let's "taco-bout" it! As a child, if I didn't like what my family prepared for dinner, I was faced with one alternative—eat a bowl of cereal. Don't like cube steak? Have Fruity Pebbles instead. A heaping bowl of artificial colors and flavors was always more appealing to me than a graying slab of meat. Right now, you might be thinking two things: *What the heck is cube steak and who feeds their child Fruity Pebbles for dinner?* I'm no therapist, but I may have just uncovered how my addiction to carbs began.

Changing my dinnertime habits was no easy task. In addition to battling my own weight demons, I had to wrestle with the demands of everyone else at the table. Whether I was preparing food for picky toddlers or my spouse on the "Eat-O" diet (meaning the "non-keto can eat anything" diet), I learned it's impossible to make everyone happy at the same time. In my experience, there are only two ways to address this situation:

1. Stop tryin' so hard. Take care of yourself and let everyone else fend for themselves. While this strategy might get Child Protective Services or a divorce lawyer involved, it is admittedly highly effective for managing what's on your plate.
2. Modify your DIRTY, LAZY, KETO recipes and/or add a starchy side dish to meet a variety of family members' needs. *Compromise.*

The dinner recipes collected here might surprise you. There are traditional favorites (like you're used to), but they have been tweaked to become "keto-fied." Sometimes, adding a sprinkle of cheese or a pad of melted butter on top of any dish *melts the heart of all critics* around your dinner table.

Recipes here won't necessarily appear to be any different from the ones you've cooked before. DIRTY, LAZY, KETO dinners don't "look" like skimpy diet dishes—they are rich and flavorful! I know this might sound shallow, but that part was important to me in my journey. I didn't want to "feel" like I was suffering. I also didn't want to deal with complaints from family members about having to eat yucky diet food. No one will suspect you are trying to lose weight with my recipes; *your secret is safe!*

Now that I am taking more chances with my cooking, I am continually surprised when I uncover new spices or flavors. I thought I hated spicy foods, but when my husband introduced me to exotic flavors from around the world such as wasabi, jalapeños, garam masala, Cajun hot sauce, and Thai-spiced coconut milk, my mind was blown! Apparently, there is a whole sixth sense out there— umami—and it has nothing to do with the Karate Kid. Do yourself a favor, and experiment with your DIRTY, LAZY, KETO cooking. *You won't be disappointed.*

VERDE CHICKEN ENCHILADAS

Verde Chicken Enchiladas are a healthier alternative to carb-laden flour tortilla–made enchiladas. Your family won't notice the difference!

2 (4.2-ounce) boneless, skinless chicken breasts, cooked

½ cup cooked, diced mushrooms

½ cup cooked, diced zucchini

8 small low-carb flour tortillas

1 cup green enchilada sauce

1 cup shredded Cheddar cheese

1 medium green onion, finely chopped

¼ cup freshly minced cilantro, divided

¼ cup sliced black olives

⅓ cup full-fat sour cream

1   Preheat oven to 350°F. Grease a 9" × 9" baking dish.

2   In a medium bowl, finely shred cooked chicken breasts. Add mushrooms and zucchini and stir to combine.

3   On a large baking sheet or clean cutting board, lay out tortillas one at a time and evenly distribute chicken and vegetable mixture in center of each tortilla. Roll each tortilla over chicken and vegetables to make tight rolls.

4   Put rolls in baking dish. Cover with green enchilada sauce and evenly top with cheese, green onion, half of the cilantro, and olives.

5   Bake 15–20 minutes until cheese melts.

6   Let cool 10 minutes. Top with sour cream and remaining cilantro and serve.

NET CARBS	
9G	

SERVES 8	
PER SERVING:	
CALORIES	200
FAT	10G
PROTEIN	15G
SODIUM	529MG
FIBER	9G
CARBOHYDRATES	18G
SUGAR	2G

TIME	
PREP TIME:	20 MIN
COOK TIME:	20 MIN

TIPS & OPTIONS

Instead of chicken, try substituting eggplant and tofu for a vegetarian-style Mexican casserole.

I like my food spicy, so I often add Cajun seasoning and chopped jalapeños.

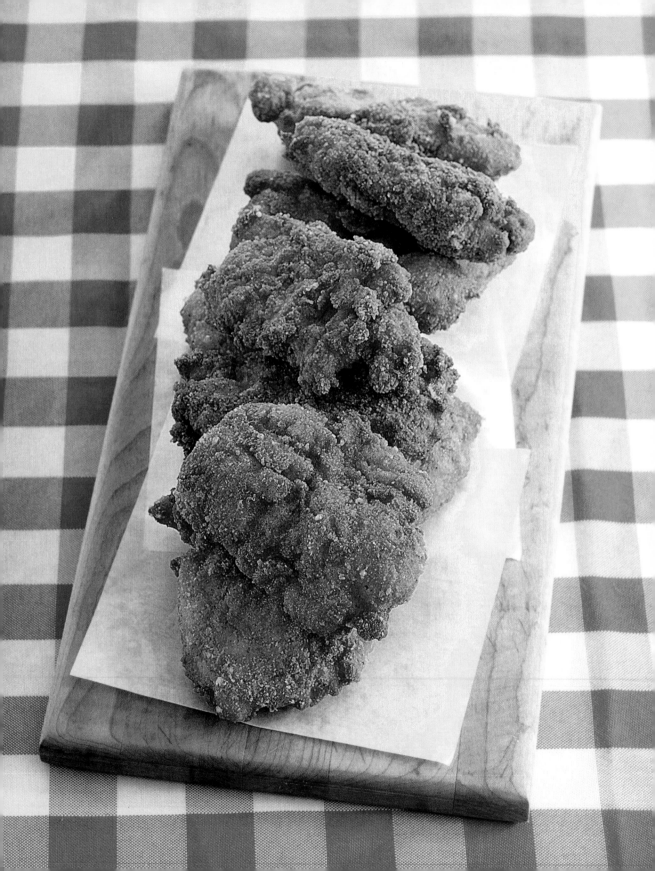

"K.F.C." KETO FRIED CHICKEN

*Nothing says comfort to me more than a bucket of fried chicken! While my drive-thru days of "finger lickin' good" might be behind me, I can still make this K.F.C. version at home. This chicken recipe is so good, your family will **seriously** think you've gone off the rails!*

1 cup vegetable oil, for frying

2 large eggs

2 tablespoons heavy whipping cream

⅔ cup blanched almond flour

⅔ cup grated Parmesan cheese

¼ teaspoon salt

½ teaspoon black pepper

½ teaspoon paprika

½ teaspoon ground cayenne

1 pound (approximately 4) boneless, skinless chicken thighs

1 In a medium pot over medium heat add vegetable oil. Make sure it is about 1" deep. Heat oil to 350°F, frequently monitoring to maintain the temperature by adjusting heat during frying.

2 In a medium bowl, add eggs and heavy whipping cream. Beat until well mixed.

3 In a separate medium bowl, add almond flour, Parmesan cheese, salt, pepper, paprika, and cayenne and mix.

4 Cut each thigh into two even pieces. If wet, pat dry.

5 Coat each piece first in the dry breading, then in the egg wash, and then the breading again.

6 Shake off any excess breading and lower the chicken into the hot oil. Fry until deep brown and cooked through, about 3–5 minutes on each side, and then drain on paper towels.

7 Repeat until all chicken is cooked. Serve right away while hot and crispy.

NET CARBS
3G

SERVES 4

PER SERVING:	
CALORIES	470
FAT	34G
PROTEIN	31G
SODIUM	507MG
FIBER	2G
CARBOHYDRATES	5G
SUGAR	1G

TIME	
PREP TIME:	15 MIN
COOK TIME:	10 MIN

TIPS & OPTIONS

Use a smaller skillet that holds two thighs at a time to cut down on oil use/waste.

Ranch dressing or sugar-free barbecue sauce make a great dip for fried chicken.

Serve with celery sticks for added crunch and to "slip in" more vegetables.

Variations for "breading mix": crushed pecans, crushed pork rinds, Parmesan cheese, soy flour, coconut flour, textured vegetable protein (TVP), or ranch powder mix.

TURKEY TACO BOATS

NET CARBS

7G

SERVES 4

PER SERVING:

CALORIES	220
FAT	9G
PROTEIN	23G
SODIUM	728MG
FIBER	3G
CARBOHYDRATES	10G
SUGAR	4G

TIME

PREP TIME:	10 MIN
COOK TIME:	30 MIN

TIPS & OPTIONS

Add cheese and sour cream if desired.

Watch out for the keto police! Some purchased taco seasoning blends contain a surprising amount of carbs. Of course, you can make your own spice blend, but honestly, who has the time? As with purchased pesto or Alfredo sauce, I've decided not to "sweat the small stuff" and occasionally indulge in buying convenience items to maintain my sanity. *Baby, I'm worth it!*

You can make these taco boats Italian-style by changing the spice blend. *Grazie!*

Tacos are a guaranteed crowd-pleaser for all ages. Because they're easy to make, inexpensive, and healthy, I find myself making Turkey Taco Boats several times a month. The varieties for tacos are endless: Lettuce wraps, cheese wraps, zucchini boats, or low-carb tortillas are just a few ideas to consider. Turkey tacos fit the needs of a versatile family. Those not eating a low-carb diet can add beans, tortillas, rice, or chips to the meal without compromising the main dish.

1 pound lean ground turkey

1 (1-ounce) package taco seasoning

¾ cup water

½ small onion, peeled and finely chopped

½ large green bell pepper, seeded and chopped

1 (4-ounce) can tomato sauce

8 large romaine lettuce leaves

1 small tomato, diced

1 In a medium pan over medium heat, brown turkey. (There shouldn't be any fat to drain.) Stir in seasoning packet and water.

2 Add onion, bell pepper, and tomato sauce to meat and stir. Cover and reduce heat to low for 15 minutes.

3 Add two lettuce "boats" per plate and fill one-eighth of the meat mixture into each boat.

4 Top with fresh tomato and serve.

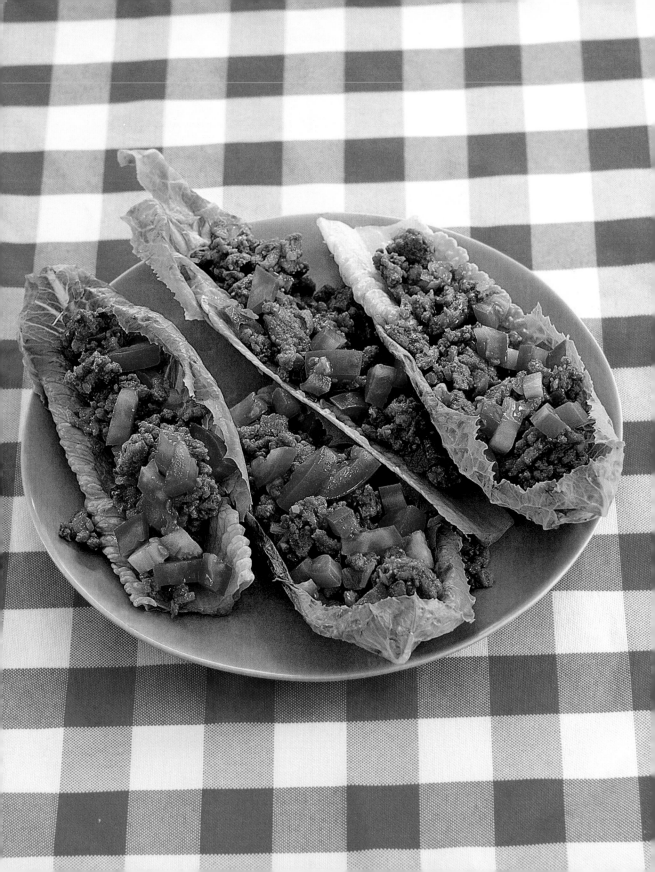

ALEX'S "CHICK AND BROCK" CASSEROLE

$ ✕

NET CARBS

8G

SERVES 8

PER SERVING:

CALORIES	427
FAT	23G
PROTEIN	31G
SODIUM	740MG
FIBER	1G
CARBOHYDRATES	9G
SUGAR	3G

TIME

PREP TIME:	10 MIN
COOK TIME:	50 MIN

TIPS & OPTIONS ⟫

In a hurry? Microwave broccoli 4–5 minutes prior to making the dish to shorten your overall bake time by 10–15 minutes.

My kids can be picky eaters. They don't like unfamiliar or complicated foods. Sometimes, I'll admit, I hide vegetables inside their foods (shhhh!), like by adding spinach to a smoothie. Interestingly, I've noticed my kids are more likely to eat a vegetable if I give it a funny name. Ever since I started calling broccoli "little trees," my children started eating it without complaining! Additionally, I've learned that adding cheese or butter to virtually any vegetable helps get it past the sniff test to everyone in my family (well maybe not the dog). Alex's "Chick and Brock" Casserole has become a family favorite; enjoy the trees, chicken, and mozzarella cheese!

1 cup heavy whipping cream

1 cup mascarpone cheese, softened

1 cup grated Parmesan cheese

3 cloves garlic, peeled and minced

2 teaspoons dried parsley

½ teaspoon salt

½ teaspoon black pepper

½ teaspoon garlic salt

1 pound cooked, shredded boneless chicken breast

4 cups raw broccoli florets

2 cups shredded whole milk mozzarella cheese, divided

1   Preheat oven to 375°F. Grease a 9" × 12" casserole dish.

2   In a large bowl, add all ingredients except chicken, broccoli, and mozzarella. Mix until blended to thick sauce.

3   In a separate large bowl, mix shredded chicken, broccoli, and 1 cup mozzarella. Add sauce mixture and mix well.

4   Transfer to casserole dish. Spread remaining 1 cup mozzarella evenly over top.

5   Bake 40–50 minutes or until broccoli is tender and cheese is golden brown.

MERRY CHRISTMAS CHICKEN

Merry Christmas Chicken earns its title by appearing only once a year in my house. My family thinks its infrequent presence is due to the red and green holiday colors, but the truth is that I dread pounding out chicken breasts to make them thinner. That's a lot of prep work, and I'm sometimes a little lazy in the kitchen! I discovered a fun hack, though, to make the job easier—instead of using a rolling pin to flatten the chicken breasts, smash the meat with the back of a cast iron pan.

4 (4.2-ounce) boneless, skinless chicken breasts

1 medium red bell pepper, seeded and chopped

1 medium green bell pepper, seeded and chopped

4 ounces full-fat cream cheese, softened

¼ teaspoon salt

¼ teaspoon black pepper

¼ teaspoon paprika

¼ teaspoon dried parsley

1 Preheat oven to 375°F.

2 Place wax paper on both sides of chicken breasts. Use a rolling pin, kitchen mallet, or cast iron skillet to pound chicken until thin (less than ¼").

3 In a medium microwave-safe bowl, microwave bell peppers 3 minutes.

4 In a separate medium bowl, mix cream cheese and softened bell peppers. Add salt and pepper.

5 Cover a large baking sheet with foil. Coat evenly with cooking spray. Lay flattened breasts on baking sheet.

6 Place one-quarter of the cream cheese mixture into the center of each pounded chicken and roll. Secure with a wet toothpick.

7 Garnish chicken with paprika and parsley to continue Christmas theme.

8 Bake 20 minutes. Serve warm.

NET CARBS	
4G	

SERVES 4	
PER SERVING:	
CALORIES	240
FAT	11G
PROTEIN	28G
SODIUM	294MG
FIBER	1G
CARBOHYDRATES	5G
SUGAR	3G

TIME	
PREP TIME:	10 MIN
COOK TIME:	23 MIN

TIPS & OPTIONS

Alternate cheeses can be substituted for equal portions of the cream cheese.

For added variety, substitute colorful vegetables like spinach or tomatoes.

Wrapping your Merry Christmas Chicken with bacon is optional, but really adds a "snap" to its presentation on the plate.

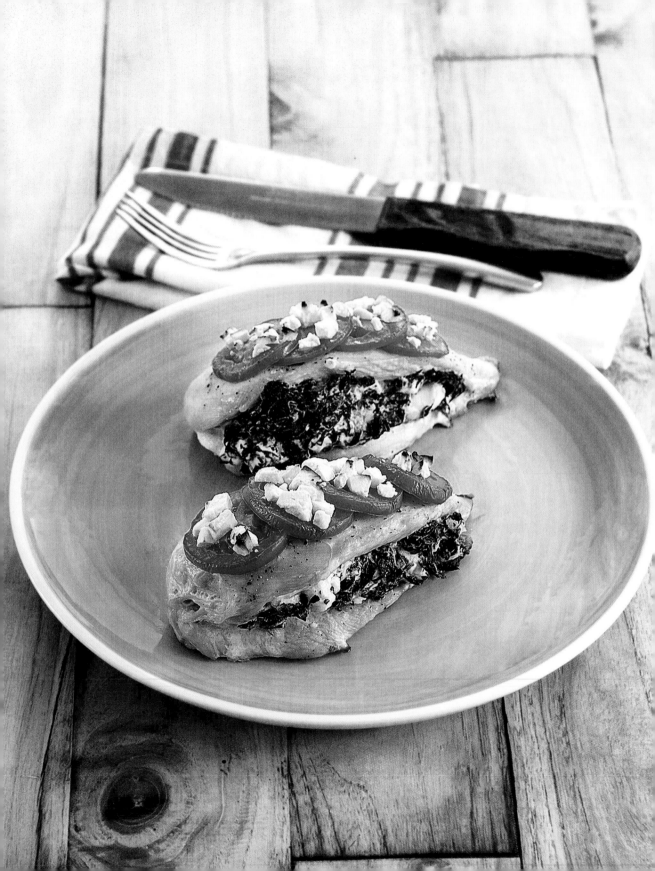

STUFFED CHICKEN FOR SUPPAH

*I get **so excited** when a dish looks as good as it tastes. Stuffed Chicken for Suppah (with spinach and feta) looks like something you would order at a five-star restaurant—the presentation is gorgeous! I highly recommend making this entrée for special occasions or when you really want to make a good impression with company.*

6 ounces chopped fresh spinach

2 cloves garlic, peeled and minced

1½ cups crumbled feta cheese, divided

2 ounces full-fat cream cheese, softened

4 (4.8-ounce) boneless, skinless chicken breasts

¼ teaspoon black pepper

2 medium Roma tomatoes, each sliced into 8 rounds

1   Preheat oven to 450°F. Line a baking sheet with parchment paper or greased foil.

2   Steam spinach in microwave 2–3 minutes (or cook in a medium skillet 3–5 minutes over medium heat). Let cooked spinach cool, then squeeze out excess moisture.

3   To a medium bowl, add spinach, garlic, and ¾ cup feta cheese.

4   Microwave cream cheese to soften for 15–30 seconds. Add to spinach mixture, stirring thoroughly.

5   Place chicken on baking sheet. Cut horizontal slit in each breast, creating a pocket. (Center your cut midway, between top and bottom of the breast.)

6   Stuff each breast with one-quarter of the total spinach mixture. Sprinkle lightly with pepper.

7   Top each breast with four tomato slices and remaining feta.

8   Bake 16–20 minutes until chicken is thoroughly cooked. Tent pan with foil if cheese starts to brown before chicken is done.

NET CARBS

5G

SERVES 4

PER SERVING:

CALORIES	364
FAT	19G
PROTEIN	40G
SODIUM	654MG
FIBER	2G
CARBOHYDRATES	7G
SUGAR	4G

TIME

PREP TIME:	10 MIN
COOK TIME:	24 MIN

TIPS & OPTIONS

Choose chicken breasts similar in size so they cook evenly in the same amount of time.

If you're on a budget, or trying to feed more guests, this same recipe can be applied to five or six smaller-sized chicken breasts. Smaller pieces also cook faster, giving you more time to socialize!

An alternate method is to quickly brown the stuffed chicken in a cast iron pan, then transfer the entire dish to the oven to bake thoroughly with the remaining cook time.

Any other type of cheese can be substituted in the same amounts.

SILKY CHICKEN WITH MUSHROOM SAUCE

Silky Chicken with Mushroom Sauce is easy, quick, and delicious! Even better, you likely have all of the ingredients for this dish in your kitchen right now. That is, of course, if you like mushrooms. Not a fan of eating fungus? Be brave, fellow ketonian, and try this recipe anyway. When I was losing weight, I surprised even myself by trying new foods. Weight loss is the best motivator for exploring new vegetables!

4 (4.2-ounce) boneless, skinless chicken breasts

4 tablespoons olive oil, divided

2 cups sliced mushrooms

½ cup diced onion

2 tablespoons unblanched almond flour

1 clove garlic, peeled and minced

½ cup half and half, divided

2 tablespoons chopped dried thyme

¼ teaspoon salt

¼ teaspoon black pepper

1 Pound chicken breasts to even thickness, about ¼" thick.

2 In a large sauté pan over medium heat, heat 2 tablespoons olive oil and then add chicken. Cook 1–2 minutes until brown on each side. Reduce heat to low.

3 Cover with secure lid and let cook additional 15 minutes (flipping at 7½ minutes). After 15 minutes, remove chicken from pan, and cover to keep warm.

4 In same pan, add mushrooms, 2 tablespoons oil, and onion. Cook over medium heat 10–15 minutes, stirring regularly. Stir in almond flour to thicken and cook an additional 2–3 minutes.

5 Add garlic, ¼ cup half and half, thyme, salt, and pepper. Keep stirring, adding more half and half if needed until the desired consistency is achieved.

6 Serve warm chicken on a plate topped with mushroom sauce.

INDOOR BBQ CHICKEN $ ✕

Every summer, when I attempt to barbecue in the backyard, I end up getting distracted by misbehaving kids throwing water balloons—then my dinner catches fire! The skin of the chicken burns so easily. My dad taught me a creative firefighting trick, however: **Pour beer over the flames!** *Because my barbecuing skills are so pathetic, I often make Indoor BBQ Chicken. It never burns and always tastes great.*

1 tablespoon sriracha sauce

2 teaspoons chili powder

2 teaspoons garlic powder

2 teaspoons onion powder

1 teaspoon salt

1 teaspoon black pepper

1 tablespoon apple cider vinegar

1 tablespoon paprika

1 (1-gram) packet 0g net carb sweetener

½ teaspoon xanthan gum

1 cup crushed tomatoes

4 medium chicken thighs with skin

1   Preheat oven to 375°F. Line a baking sheet with parchment paper or greased foil.

2   In a small saucepan over medium-high heat, make the barbecue sauce by mixing all the ingredients except the chicken and bring to boil. Let simmer 5 minutes, stirring regularly.

3   Using a basting brush, apply about half the barbecue sauce to both sides of thighs. Place chicken on baking sheet.

4   Cook 20 minutes. Flip chicken and reapply remaining sauce. Cook another 20 minutes until chicken is thoroughly cooked.

5   Serve warm or cold.

NET CARBS

7G

SERVES 4

PER SERVING:

CALORIES	362
FAT	19G
PROTEIN	34G
SODIUM	951MG
FIBER	3G
CARBOHYDRATES	10G
SUGAR	4G

TIME

PREP TIME:	10 MIN
COOK TIME:	45 MIN

TIPS & OPTIONS

If you have the extra time and prefer really moist chicken, "poach" the meat before starting this recipe. Boiling the chicken thighs for 7–10 minutes or boneless and skinless breasts for 10–15 minutes really plumps them up and adds flavor! This can be done ahead of time, like the night before. Store the poached chicken in the fridge until you are ready to use in this recipe.

To turn up the heat, add ½ teaspoon cayenne pepper to your sauce.

CHIPOTLE CHICKEN FAJITA BOWL $ ✕

NET CARBS

8G

SERVES 4

PER SERVING:

CALORIES	610
FAT	40G
PROTEIN	39G
SODIUM	660MG
FIBER	8G
CARBOHYDRATES	16G
SUGAR	5G

TIME

PREP TIME:	10 MIN
COOK TIME:	30 MIN

TIPS & OPTIONS 〉〉

Missing beans? This recipe pairs well with a serving of low-carb black soybeans (cans ordered online). They contain only 1 gram of net carbs per half cup—AMAZING!

Try shrimp or tilapia instead of chicken!

If you have a vegetarian or vegan in the family, cook the meat separately.

If your family loves Mexican food as much as mine does, this meal is sure to become an instant hit. It's like eating at Chipotle Mexican Grill, but without leaving the house! My non-keto family members make their own sides of rice, beans, or tortillas to add to their meal without disrupting the main dish. Everyone's happy with the Chipotle Chicken Fajita Bowl.

3 tablespoons unsalted butter

1½ pounds boneless, skinless chicken thighs, cut into thin strips

¼ teaspoon salt

1 small yellow onion, peeled and diced

1 large green bell pepper, seeded and diced

2 tablespoons taco seasoning

6 cups chopped romaine lettuce

1 cup shredded Mexican cheese

½ cup full-fat sour cream

2 large avocados, peeled, pitted, and diced

1 small tomato, chopped

4 tablespoons finely chopped cilantro

1   In a large skillet over medium heat, add butter and fry chicken for 5 minutes while stirring just to brown. Season chicken with salt. Sauté 10–15 minutes, stirring regularly.

2   Add onion, bell pepper, and taco seasoning. Reduce heat to low and cook 7–10 minutes. Stir often until vegetables have softened.

3   Distribute lettuce evenly to serving bowls, then add cooked chicken and vegetables. Top with cheese, sour cream, diced avocados, tomato, and cilantro.

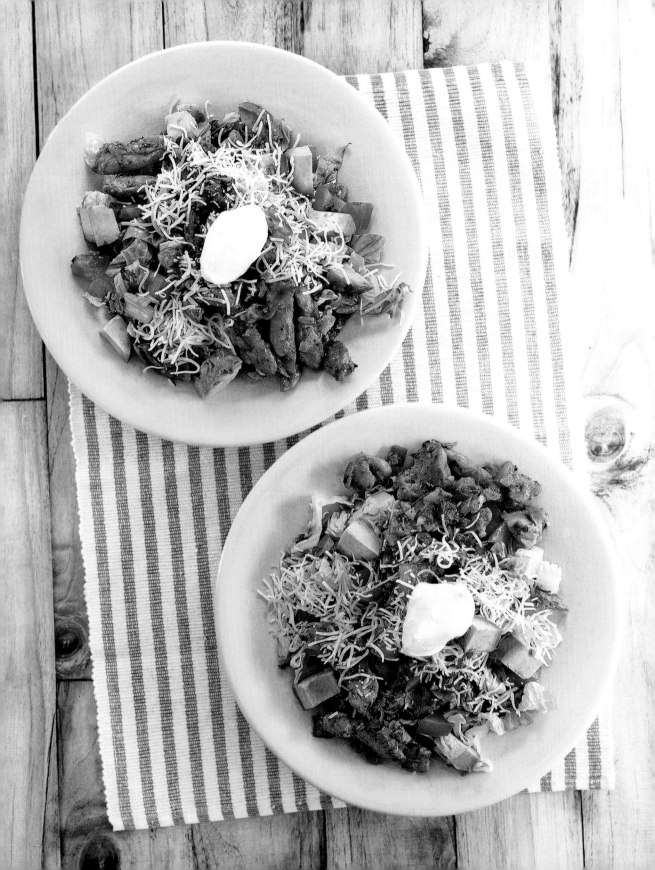

FLUFFY CHICKEN

TIPS & OPTIONS

Complement this dish with a bagged salad mix and your dinner duties are done.

I highly recommend that you double the recipe to ensure there are leftovers, as you will definitely be craving Fluffy Chicken tomorrow!

If your family is anything like mine, Fluffy Chicken will become one of your most requested dishes. With just five minutes of prep time, it will become your favorite too!

½ cup chicken broth

1 (1-ounce) package ranch powder seasoning mix

2 pounds boneless, skinless chicken breasts

8 ounces full-fat cream cheese, softened

8 slices no-sugar-added bacon, cooked and crumbled

½ cup shredded Cheddar cheese

1 Add chicken broth to slow cooker and stir in ranch powder seasoning packet.

2 Add chicken and cover. Cook 2 hours 45 minutes on high or 5 hours 15 minutes on low.

3 Remove lid. Drain excess broth, leaving around ½ cup for moisture depending on preference.

4 Shred chicken.

5 In a small microwave-safe bowl, microwave cream cheese 20–30 seconds. Combine with crumbled bacon and Cheddar cheese.

6 Add cream cheese mixture to shredded chicken. Cover and heat 10 minutes on high temperature until cheeses melt. Serve warm.

N'AWLINS CHICKEN

One of my happiest memories with my husband is when we joined a wedding parade in New Orleans. With a police escort and live jazz band, we waltzed down Bourbon Street wearing our festive beads. Every time I make N'awlins Chicken, I think back to our many trips to the magical city where we eloped.

1 teaspoon olive oil

2 pounds boneless, skinless chicken thighs

¼ teaspoon salt

⅛ teaspoon black pepper

3 tablespoons unsalted butter

¼ cup minced onion

3 cloves garlic, peeled and minced

1 cup bourbon

2 cups chicken stock

1   In a large saucepan over medium heat, heat olive oil, then add chicken thighs. Season with salt and pepper and sear 3 minutes on each side until golden brown.

2   Add butter, onion, and garlic, and sauté until the onion and garlic are brown (3–5 minutes).

3   Pour bourbon and chicken stock over chicken and boil.

4   Reduce heat to medium and cook 25–30 minutes, flipping chicken halfway through.

5   Cool and serve chicken with bourbon sauce.

NET CARBS

4G

SERVES 6

PER SERVING:

CALORIES	391
FAT	18G
PROTEIN	40G
SODIUM	372MG
FIBER	0G
CARBOHYDRATES	4G
SUGAR	2G

TIME

PREP TIME:	10 MIN
COOK TIME:	41 MIN

TIPS & OPTIONS

Serve this dish over a bed of shredded lettuce or riced cauliflower.

A great side to consider would be the Get Loaded Smashed Cauliflower (see recipe in Chapter 7).

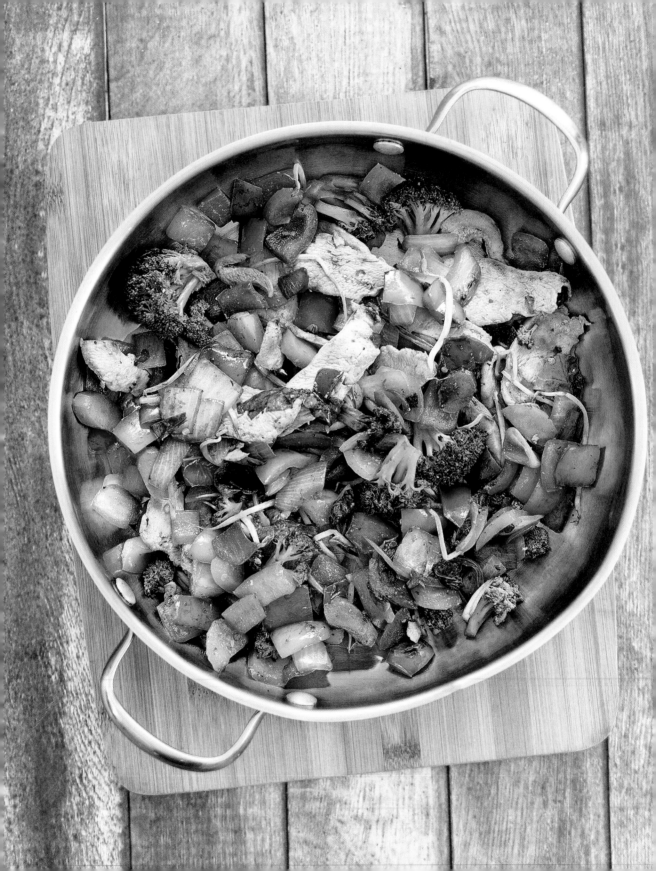

WOK THIS WAY ✕ 🍲

*Growing up, my dad frequently made stir-fry for dinner. His signature ingredient was canned pineapple—**yuck!** To this day, I can't think about stir-fry without tasting phantom sweet-and-salty flavors. Now that I have my own family, I've instituted an official "no pineapple policy" for stir-fry. I wash and cut up a million other ingredients, though. Yes, it's a lot of work to prep the assorted meats and vegetables, but the end product is absolutely satisfying. Each person in my family assembles their own bowl—stir-fry is the personalized pizza of Asian food. To make this easier, I heat up four skillets on the stove.*

2 tablespoons sesame oil

2 (4.8-ounce) boneless, skinless chicken breasts, thinly cut

½ tablespoon ground ginger

1 large green bell pepper, seeded and chopped

1 medium yellow bell pepper, seeded and chopped

1 small red bell pepper, seeded and chopped

1 small carrot, peeled and sliced

1 cup cut bean sprouts, 2" sections

1 cup broccoli florets

2 cups chopped fresh spinach

1 small white onion, peeled and diced

2 cloves garlic, peeled and minced

1 tablespoon soy sauce

¼ teaspoon chili pepper flakes

1 Heat a large skillet over medium heat and add sesame oil. Add chicken and ginger and partially cook 10 minutes, stirring regularly. Remove chicken and set aside.

2 Add bell peppers, carrot, bean sprouts, broccoli, spinach, onion, and garlic to hot skillet and sauté with lid off 15–20 minutes until softened, stirring regularly.

3 Return chicken to skillet for 15 minutes. Stir in soy sauce and chili flakes.

4 Turn off the heat and serve warm.

NET CARBS

9G

SERVES 4

PER SERVING:

CALORIES	174
FAT	8G
PROTEIN	14G
SODIUM	304MG
FIBER	3G
CARBOHYDRATES	12G
SUGAR	4G

TIME

PREP TIME:	15 MIN
COOK TIME:	45 MIN

TIPS & OPTIONS

Any low-carb vegetables can be added to this recipe. Be creative!

Shrimp, pork, beef, peanuts, egg, and tofu also make great stir-fry proteins.

To ensure the tougher vegetables cook properly (broccoli, carrots), I cut them into smaller pieces and precook them a bit in the microwave.

Omit the chili pepper flakes if you are not a fan of spicy food.

Feeling adventurous? Add additional vegetables, but please, I beg you, leave out the canned pineapple.

FOUR HORSEMEN BUTTER CHICKEN

NET CARBS

7G

SERVES 8

PER SERVING:

CALORIES	298
FAT	16G
PROTEIN	30G
SODIUM	729MG
FIBER	1G
CARBOHYDRATES	8G
SUGAR	2G

TIME

PREP TIME:	10 MIN
COOK TIME:	27 MIN

TIPS & OPTIONS

A great side dish for this recipe is plain steamed cauliflower. Serve Four Horsemen Butter Chicken on top of the cauliflower in place of rice.

Other rice or naan alternatives include "zoodles," or zucchini noodles, or even simpler, a bed of lettuce.

If the stores in your area don't sell Indian spices, order them online. Garam masala will last for years in your spice rack.

Lastly, in case you feel like "skipping a few steps," I won't tell anyone if you buy an Indian "starter sauce" at the grocery store (located in the ethnic foods aisle). *This is our little secret, by the way!*

The adults in our home absolutely LOVE Indian food. We make Four Horsemen Butter Chicken as often as we can. Even my teenage daughter has fallen in love with Indian flavors. This recipe is a bit more complicated (and has more ingredients) than many of the recipes in this cookbook, but the final result makes your efforts worthwhile. With the "four horsemen" of Indian spices in your cupboard—garam masala, coriander, curry powder, and turmeric— an entire continent of recipes will be at your fingertips.

1 tablespoon unsalted butter

1 tablespoon olive oil

1 medium onion, peeled and diced

3 cloves garlic, peeled and minced

2 teaspoons peeled and grated fresh ginger

2 pounds boneless, skinless chicken breasts, cooked and cut into ¾" chunks

3 ounces tomato paste

3 ounces red curry paste

1 tablespoon garam masala

1 teaspoon chili powder

1 teaspoon mustard seeds

1 teaspoon ground coriander

1 teaspoon curry

1 teaspoon salt

⅛ teaspoon black pepper

1 (14-ounce) can unsweetened coconut milk

1 teaspoon chopped cilantro

1 In a large skillet over medium-high heat, heat butter and olive oil. Add onion and fry until soft, about 3–5 minutes. Mix in garlic and ginger. Cook 1–2 minutes more.

2 Add cooked chicken to skillet. Add tomato paste, red curry paste, garam masala, chili powder, mustard seeds, coriander, and curry. Add salt and pepper. Stir until well mixed and chicken cubes are well coated.

3 Stir in coconut milk and bring to boil. Reduce heat. Cover and simmer 20 minutes.

4 Remove from heat. Let cool 10 minutes and serve warm with cilantro sprinkled on top.

INFERNO TANDOORI CHICKEN

*While you likely don't have a 500°F kiln in your kitchen, you certainly have large Ziploc bags and full-fat plain yogurt in your fridge. The trick to enjoying Inferno Tandoori Chicken is patience and planning. To ensure the strongest flavors while creating bold, brilliant color in your dish, marinate your chicken with yogurt sauce **at least** an hour, but preferably overnight.*

2 teaspoons paprika

2 teaspoons ginger paste

1 teaspoon ground coriander

1 teaspoon ground cumin

1 teaspoon garam masala

1 teaspoon ground cayenne

1 cup plain whole milk Greek yogurt

4 (4.2-ounce) boneless, skinless chicken breasts

1 In a medium bowl, mix together all spices. Add yogurt, stirring to blend thoroughly.

2 Using a spatula, scoop yogurt mixture into a gallon-sized Ziploc bag.

3 Cut each chicken breast into four strips.

4 Transfer chicken to marinate in yogurt mixture, sealing bag and carefully kneading through the plastic bag, ensuring chicken is completely covered with sauce.

5 Let sit in refrigerator for at least 1 hour (but preferably overnight).

6 Preheat oven to 400°F. Line a baking sheet with parchment paper.

7 Remove chicken pieces from the bag and place onto baking sheet, trying to keep as much of the sauce as possible that clings to the meat. Don't add any extra sauce from the bag. Bake 40–45 minutes or until fully cooked, flipping once at 20 minutes.

8 Remove from the oven and serve warm.

NET CARBS
2G

SERVES 4	
PER SERVING:	
CALORIES	189
FAT	5G
PROTEIN	33G
SODIUM	65MG
FIBER	1G
CARBOHYDRATES	3G
SUGAR	2G

TIME	
PREP TIME:	1 HR TO
	OVERNIGHT
COOK TIME:	45 MIN

TIPS & OPTIONS

Salmon can be substituted, though with a reduction in cook time (based on thickness).

Beef and pork can also be substituted, but the brilliant orange/red color of the sauce will not be as impressive since those meats are darker than chicken.

Serve Inferno Tandoori Chicken on top of steamed cauliflower or a bed of shredded lettuce.

STEPH'S STUFFED PEPPERS

TIPS & OPTIONS

Add more toppings if you are adventurous: Diced jalapeños, avocado, sour cream, or diced green onions would all be great.

Microwaving the raw unstuffed bell peppers for a few minutes will soften them up a bit and ensure the dish will cook completely in the oven.

*When bell peppers are in season, Steph's Stuffed Peppers recipe becomes more affordable—**those peppers can get pricey!** Using all three colors of bell peppers makes the dish look more festive, but keep in mind that the green bell peppers contain the least amount of carbs of all the colored peppers. This is a fun recipe for the holiday season too—nothing says "Merry Christmas" like red and green bell peppers.*

4 medium green bell peppers, seeded

1 medium red bell pepper, seeded

1 medium yellow bell pepper, seeded

1 pound lean ground turkey

1 cup cooked riced cauliflower

¾ cup no-sugar-added salsa

1 teaspoon chili powder

1 teaspoon ground cumin

½ teaspoon black pepper

¼ teaspoon salt

1 cup shredded Cheddar cheese

1 Preheat oven to 375°F. Grease a 9" × 13" baking dish.

2 Remove stems from peppers by cutting tight circle around stem. Cut peppers in half vertically from stem to bottom. Remove the seeds and membranes from insides. Wash gently and pat dry.

3 In a medium skillet over medium-high heat, cook ground turkey, stirring regularly, about 10 minutes.

4 Add riced cauliflower. Stir in salsa and spices.

5 Arrange bell pepper halves open-side up in baking dish. Fill each pepper half with one-twelfth of meat mixture and top with cheese.

6 Bake 30 minutes, or until peppers are softened and cheese is fully melted. Remove from oven and let cool. Serve warm.

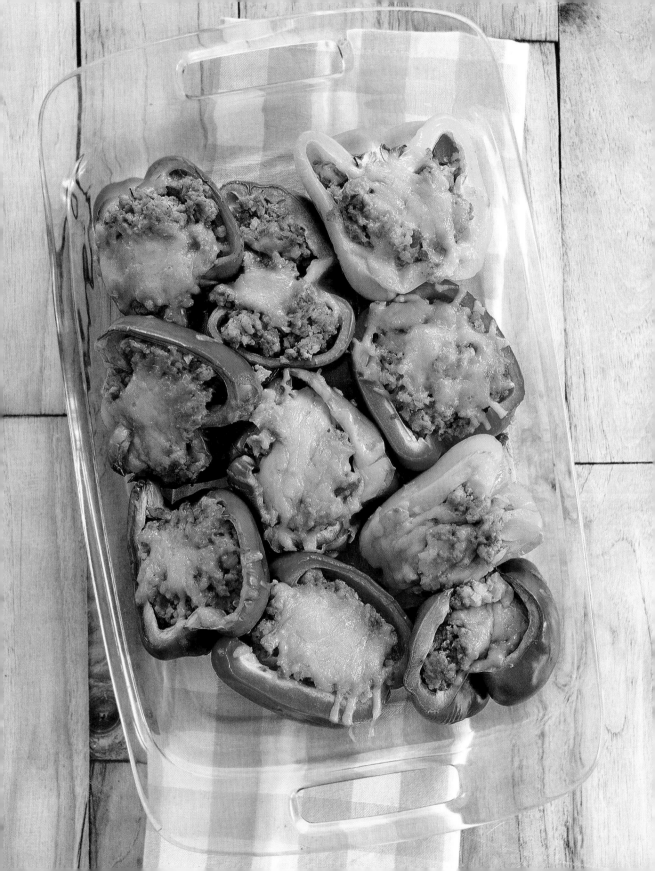

DRUNKEN POT ROAST

TIPS & OPTIONS

I recommend Get Loaded Smashed Cauliflower (see recipe in Chapter 7) as an excellent side dish with this meal. Pour "gravy" from the slow cooker onto your "faux" mashed potatoes.

"Roast" is a general term that can apply to a number of cuts of beef: top sirloin, top round, bottom round, etc. Basically, any thick cut of beef that could benefit from the tenderizing effects of the slow cooker.

This lazy, yet hearty meal is best enjoyed during the winter months with a fire going and a new Netflix series ready to watch. It's so easy to make, with only five ingredients and five minutes of prep time. By the time you finish binge-watching an entire season, Drunken Pot Roast will be finished cooking in the slow cooker and your house will smell amazing.

1 (4-pound) roast
1 (1-ounce) package ranch dressing mix
1 cup chopped celery
½ cup unsalted butter, softened
1 (12-ounce) can low-carb beer

1 Place roast in slow cooker and cover with dressing mix, celery, butter, and beer.

2 Cover and cook on low heat for 8 hours.

3 After cooking is finished, let roast sit 15 minutes. Carve and serve warm.

LAZY MEATLOAF

Meatloaf wasn't my childhood favorite meal until I learned I could decorate it like a cake, "icing" the meatloaf with a thick layer of mashed potatoes and cheese. Icing the meatloaf made it look quite fancy; well-presented food tends to taste better, in my opinion. This Lazy Meatloaf recipe mimics the recipe I grew up with in Michigan. You will quickly see the appeal of this tasty dish—it's fast to prepare and looks super impressive after it's "decorated." Check out my special presentation in the Tips and Options section.

5 tablespoons no-sugar-added ketchup, divided

1½ pounds lean ground beef

2 large eggs

½ cup crushed pork rinds

1 small white onion, peeled and chopped

1 tablespoon Italian seasoning

1 teaspoon mustard powder

1 teaspoon soy sauce

½ teaspoon minced garlic

½ teaspoon black pepper

1 Preheat oven to 400°F. Grease a 9" × 5" × 2½" loaf pan.

2 In a large bowl, combine 3 tablespoons ketchup with all remaining ingredients until combined.

3 Add the mixture to the prepared pan. Top with remaining ketchup and cover with foil.

4 Bake 50–60 minutes. Serve warm.

NET CARBS
2G

SERVES 6

PER SERVING:

CALORIES	278
FAT	14G
PROTEIN	30G
SODIUM	450MG
FIBER	0G
CARBOHYDRATES	2G
SUGAR	1G

TIME

PREP TIME:	15 MIN
COOK TIME:	60 MIN

TIPS & OPTIONS

Ground turkey or lean ground pork can easily be substituted for ground beef in this recipe.

To improve the presentation of your meatloaf, "ice" it like a cake using warmed Get Loaded Smashed Cauliflower (see recipe in Chapter 7). Then, sprinkle shredded cheese over the iced meatloaf and melt the cheese under a broiler just prior to serving.

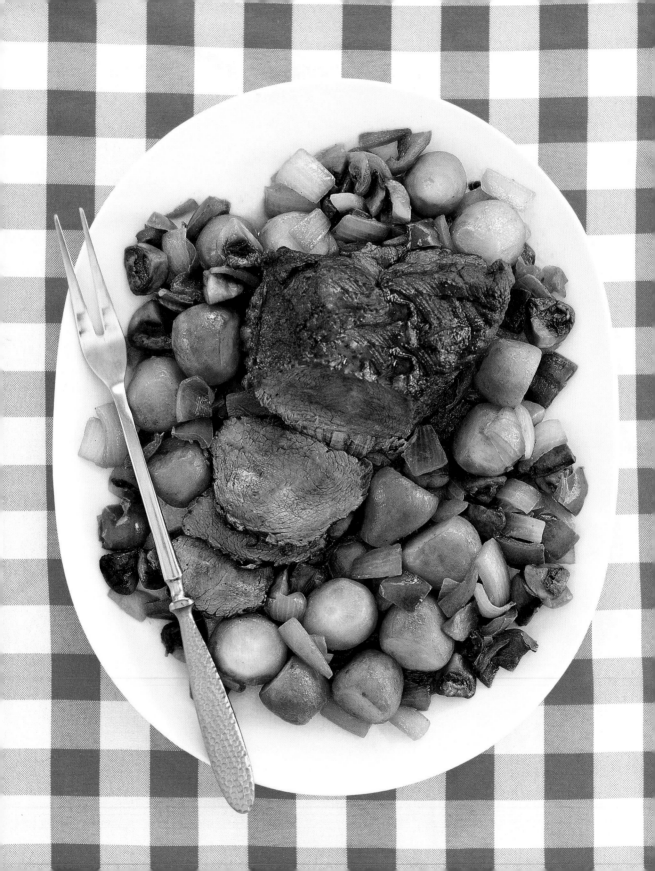

HILLBILLY POT ROAST WITH "TATERS"

Coming from the Midwest, my family ate a steady diet of "meat-n-taters" for dinner. Today, my version of "taters" involves the most surprising keto hack: radishes. Yes, radishes! They taste and even look similar to boiled cooked potatoes when steamed in a pressure cooker.

2 tablespoons avocado oil, divided

8 ounces sliced white mushrooms

2 medium green bell peppers, seeded and chopped

16 ounces radishes, trimmed

1 medium onion, peeled and chopped

2 cloves garlic, peeled and minced

1 teaspoon salt

1 teaspoon black pepper

1 (2-pound) roast

1 cup beef stock

2 tablespoons Worcestershire sauce

NET CARBS

8G

SERVES 6

PER SERVING:

CALORIES	371
FAT	20G
PROTEIN	35G
SODIUM	654MG
FIBER	2G
CARBOHYDRATES	10G
SUGAR	4G

TIME

PREP TIME:	20 MIN
COOK TIME:	75 MIN

1 Press Sauté button on your Instant Pot® and set timer for 15 minutes. Heat 1 tablespoon oil in pot and add mushrooms, bell peppers, radishes, onion, and garlic. Sauté vegetables and stir until onions are caramelized (with lid off), about 10–15 minutes. Note that radishes will not be fully cooked.

2 Remove veggies and add remaining 1 tablespoon oil into the Instant Pot®. Sprinkle salt and pepper on all sides of roast and place into Instant Pot®. Press Sauté button and set timer for 10 minutes. Brown meat on each side 5 minutes, leaving lid off.

3 Remove roast and return metal grate to base of Instant Pot®. Set roast on the grate. Pour stock and Worcestershire sauce over meat. Secure lid and press the Pressure Cooker button. Set high pressure setting to 45 minutes.

4 After 45 minutes, use quick pressure release, then remove lid.

5 Add vegetable mix back to the Instant Pot®. Secure lid and select Pressure Cooker setting for 5 minutes on high pressure. (Note, the vegetables will cook while it takes the Instant Pot® 5–10 minutes to get up to the right pressure before the timer starts.) When the timer goes off, use the quick pressure release.

6 Let the roast and the veggies sit in the Instant Pot® 5 minutes before serving.

TIPS & OPTIONS

Save time by purchasing prewashed and pre-sliced mushrooms.

Radishes stay fresh for long periods of time in the crisper drawer of your refrigerator. Stock up on bags of radishes to keep on hand when a craving for potatoes strikes.

"Roast" is a general term that can apply to a number of cuts of beef: top sirloin, top round, bottom round, etc. Basically, any thick cut of beef that could benefit from the tenderizing effects of the pressure cooker.

For variety, I often enjoy topping my cooked radishes with sour cream, shredded cheese, and bacon bits.

OPEN SESAME MEATBALLS ✕

I'm always surprised by how much my kids love meatballs. My son, who basically hates all protein, pops these in his mouth like McDonald's chicken nuggets. I've learned that appearances really do matter when it comes to serving meatballs. If the meatballs are uniform in size and shape, my family wolfs them down before I've even sat down to join them for dinner.

Meatballs

3 teaspoons sesame oil, divided

2 large eggs

1 pound lean ground turkey

2 medium green onions, finely chopped

1 cup finely shredded green cabbage

2 teaspoons soy sauce

2 teaspoons peeled and grated fresh ginger

1 clove garlic, peeled and minced

2 tablespoons flaxseed meal

⅛ teaspoon black pepper

Lettuce Boats

8 leaves romaine lettuce, large enough to be "boats"

1 small red bell pepper, seeded and sliced

1 small cucumber, peeled and thinly sliced into half-moons

Sauce

¼ cup soy sauce

1 packet 0g net carb sweetener

2 tablespoons water

¼ teaspoon sesame oil

⅛ teaspoon red pepper flakes

1. In a large bowl, mix 1 teaspoon oil with all remaining meatball ingredients.

2. Form mixture into 2"-sized uniform meatballs.

3. In a large skillet over medium heat, heat remaining 2 teaspoons oil and fully cook meatballs on all sides (20–30 minutes total), turning fragile meatballs GENTLY using tongs.

4. On a large platter, arrange romaine lettuce leaves along with decorative bell pepper and cucumber slices.

5. In a small bowl, combine sauce ingredients.

6. Transfer meatballs to lettuce "boats" (approximately one per boat). Serve lettuce boats with the sauce on the side in four small dipping bowls.

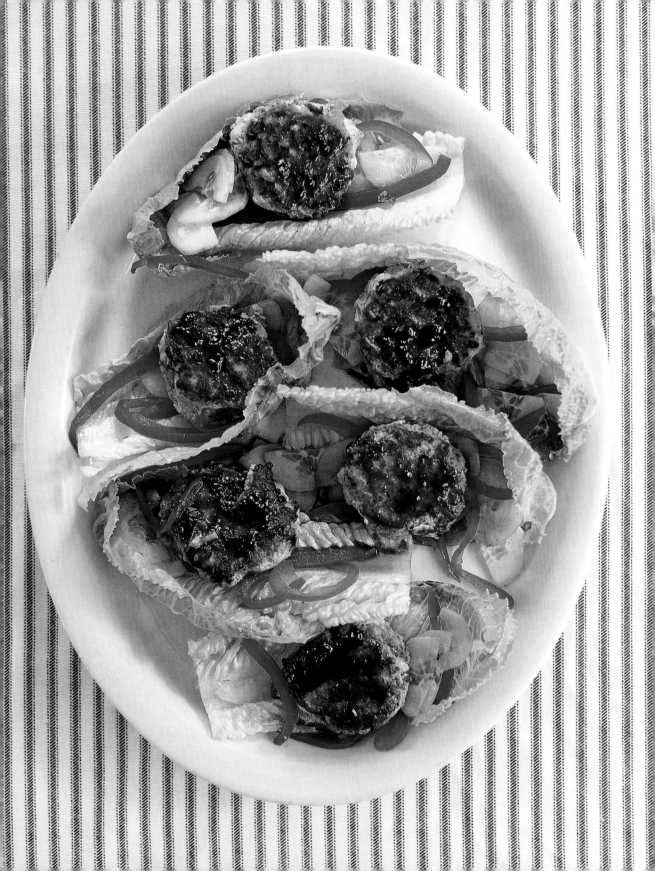

LEMON AND DILL SALMON KABOBS

SERVES 8

PER SERVING:

CALORIES	137
FAT	8G
PROTEIN	12G
SODIUM	117MG
FIBER	0G
CARBOHYDRATES	1G
SUGAR	1G

TIME

PREP TIME:	10 MIN
COOK TIME:	15 MIN

TIPS & OPTIONS

When the weather is bad, making barbecuing impossible, I sometimes bake my kabobs in the toaster oven.

For variety, add additional low-carb vegetables or other meats to your skewers. Examples include shrimp, chicken, beef, bell peppers, tomatoes, mushrooms, broccoli, red onion, and eggplant.

My children love to make kabobs. I find they are more likely to eat vegetables when they choose which vegetables to add to their personalized skewers. I'm often surprised (*and impressed!*) by their brave little choices.

Since it offers so many health benefits, I strive to eat more salmon. The healthy fats inside this oily fish are perfect for DIRTY, LAZY, KETO. Cooking salmon on the grill makes cleanup a snap and prevents my house from becoming too stinky! Even my kids have been known to eat "pink chicken" **as they are confused about what I'm serving them.** *Please don't tell my children that salmon is not from a chicken!*

1 tablespoon fresh dill

¼ cup olive oil

¼ cup lemon juice

¼ teaspoon salt

¼ teaspoon black pepper

⅛ teaspoon ground cayenne

1 pound salmon, cubed

1 medium zucchini, sliced into ¼" rounds

1. Soak wooden skewers in water for at least 5 minutes in a shallow dish to prevent them from burning on grill.

2. In a medium bowl, combine dill, oil, lemon juice, salt, pepper, and cayenne.

3. Toss salmon cubes with marinade and stir to coat completely. Let marinate 10 minutes while prepping grill.

4. Clean and grease outdoor grill grate. Preheat outdoor grill to medium heat for 5 minutes.

5. Skewer salmon and zucchini on eight skewers using alternating pattern. Brush with remaining marinade.

6. Grill kabobs ½" apart, turning regularly until fully cooked, about 15 minutes total cooking time.

SWEDISH BIKINI TEAM MEATBALLS

*My Scandinavian roots might be obvious to you with my light blue eyes and blonde (albeit from a bottle) hair. Other than my appearance, I don't retain a lot of culture from my heritage. This DIRTY, LAZY, KETO Swedish Bikini Team Meatballs recipe attempts to honor my roots and will help keep me wearing a bikini this summer (**stretch marks, loose skin, and all!**). The name of this dish is an homage to the beer commercials of the '90s featuring the Swedish Bikini Team.*

2 tablespoons unsalted butter, softened

⅓ cup diced onion

½ teaspoon allspice

3 cloves garlic, peeled and minced

1½ pounds ground beef

¼ cup half and half

1 large egg

1 cup pork rinds, crushed

2 teaspoons Worcestershire sauce, divided

¼ teaspoon salt

¼ teaspoon black pepper

1 cup beef broth

1 cup heavy whipping cream

1 teaspoon xanthan gum

1. In a small skillet over medium heat, melt butter. Add onion and sauté 5 minutes until onion is translucent. Add allspice and garlic. Cook another minute. Remove from the heat.

2. In a large mixing bowl, combine ground beef, half and half, egg, pork rinds, 1 teaspoon Worcestershire sauce, onion mixture, salt, and pepper. Combine well and form into 2"-sized balls.

3. Add balls to slow cooker and pour beef broth over them. Cook on high 3 hours (or low 6 hours).

4. Remove balls from slow cooker with tongs and set aside.

5. Add cream, xanthan gum, and remaining Worcestershire sauce to liquid in slow cooker. Stir well and let thicken 5–10 minutes. Add meatballs back into slow cooker just to cover with the sauce.

6. Serve meatballs with the white sauce.

TIPS & OPTIONS

If not using a lean meat, I prefer to drain most of the fat from the bottom of the slow cooker right after the cooked meatballs are removed. Don't worry; there is still plenty of fat inside the meatballs. Replace with water to ensure you have plenty of gravy.

I recommend serving this dish with well-cooked radishes, a delicious potato substitute!

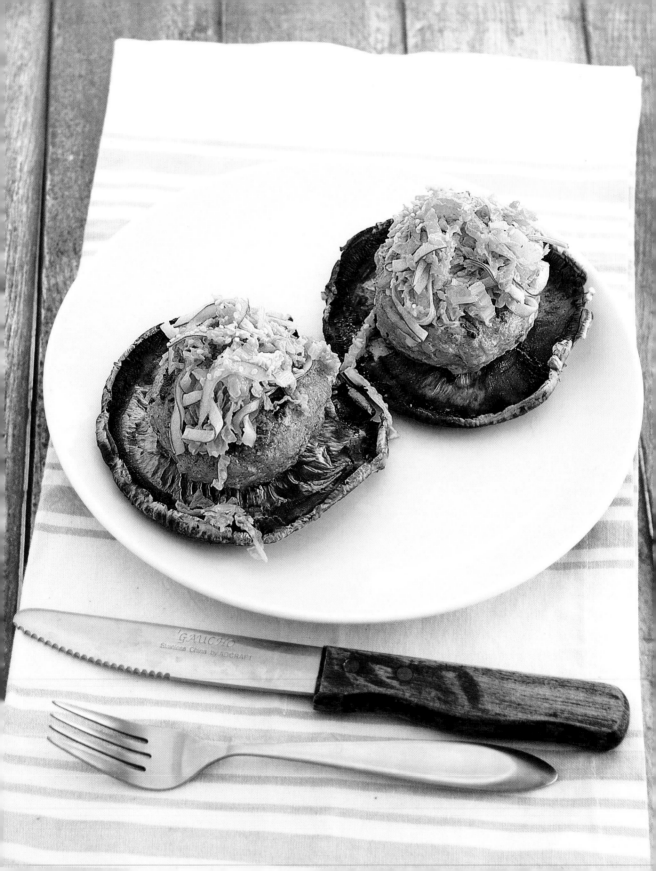

TOPLESS BURGERS

When my son was little, he accidentally ordered a "topless burger" (instead of requesting a burger patty without the bun). The waitress had a good laugh! Ever since then, my family refers to bunless burgers as "topless."

1 pound lean ground turkey

¼ cup finely chopped green apple

1 tablespoon ground ginger

2 (1-gram) packets 0g net carb sweetener

1 tablespoon soy sauce

4 large whole portabella mushroom caps

2 tablespoons sesame oil

¼ small red onion, peeled and thinly sliced

4 tablespoons full-fat mayonnaise

2 cups shredded cabbage

1 tablespoon sesame seeds

1. In a large bowl, mix ground turkey with apple, ginger, sweetener, and soy sauce. Form mixture into four equal bun-sized patties.

2. Brush portabella mushroom caps with sesame oil.

3. On clean, prepped grill, cook burgers and portabella mushroom caps over medium flame, 5–7 minutes on each side, until desired level of cooking. Be very gentle flipping the mushroom caps.

4. Remove from flame and assemble Topless Burgers with portabella mushroom underneath burger patty.

5. Serve with onion, mayonnaise, cabbage, and sesame seeds.

NET CARBS	
5G	

SERVES 4	
PER SERVING:	
CALORIES	393
FAT	27G
PROTEIN	27G
SODIUM	403MG
FIBER	3G
CARBOHYDRATES	8G
SUGAR	4G

TIME	
PREP TIME:	10 MIN
COOK TIME:	14 MIN

TIPS & OPTIONS

For added spice, include red pepper flakes on your Topless Burgers.

Add cheese if desired. Get crazy and grill onions or sliced mushrooms as toppings if you have them available.

BASIL COCONUT CURRY SHRIMP

Thai food earns runner-up status for best foreign food (behind Indian, of course). The coconut milk and fresh basil tastes delight my bland Midwestern palate. Because Thai restaurants often use sweetened coconut milk in their curry recipes, I was all the more motivated to re-create a DIRTY, LAZY, KETO version at home. You will enjoy this simple basil dish and be surprised by the rich flavor.

TIPS & OPTIONS

Serve on a bed of steamed cauliflower, eggplant, shredded lettuce, or "zoodles" instead of rice. Zoodles are strips of zucchini sautéed lightly to resemble noodles. You can purchase zoodles fresh or frozen, or even make your own. (Oxo sells an inexpensive hand tool that shreds zucchini into long, noodle-like strips.)

Chicken may be substituted for shrimp.

1 tablespoon coconut oil

16 ounces prepared medium shrimp

¼ teaspoon salt

⅛ teaspoon black pepper

⅔ medium red bell pepper, seeded and sliced

½ medium green bell pepper, seeded and sliced

½ medium onion, peeled and sliced

¾ tablespoon minced garlic

1 tablespoon ground ginger

1½ tablespoons red curry paste

1 (14-ounce) can unsweetened coconut milk

½ cup finely chopped fresh basil

1 In a deep medium pan over medium-high heat, melt coconut oil. Add shrimp to pan and season with salt and pepper while stirring 5–10 minutes until shrimp turns pink. Remove shrimp from pan.

2 Add bell peppers and onion. Sauté 5 minutes until softened. Add garlic and ginger with curry paste and stir to coat vegetables. Return cooked shrimp to pan.

3 Stir in coconut milk and fresh basil. Mix well. Cover and reduce heat to medium-low and simmer 10–15 minutes, stirring regularly.

4 Remove from heat, let cool, and serve.

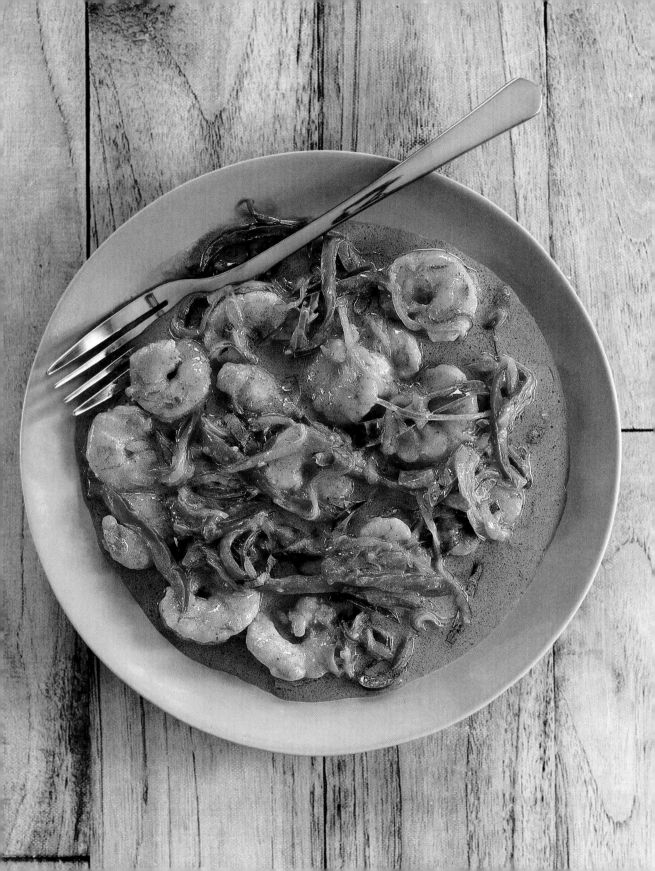

MUFFIN TOP TUNA POPS $ ✕

NET CARBS

1G

SERVES 6

PER SERVING:

CALORIES	275
FAT	22G
PROTEIN	14G
SODIUM	483MG
FIBER	0G
CARBOHYDRATES	1G
SUGAR	1G

TIME

PREP TIME:	10 MIN
COOK TIME:	25 MIN

TIPS & OPTIONS ⟫

The tuna mix will rise some during the baking process so be careful not to overfill the muffin cups.

Sometimes I substitute more of the tuna for either of the cheeses for a meatier muffin.

Anything that resembles a muffin appeals to me! Because canned tuna is an inexpensive staple, I keep plenty on hand (along with frozen riced cauliflower, frozen chicken breasts, frozen ground turkey, and tofu blocks). I like sneaking more protein into my diet with this bite-sized snack.

1 (5-ounce) can tuna in water, drained

2 large eggs

¾ cup shredded Cheddar cheese

¾ cup shredded pepper jack cheese

¼ cup full-fat sour cream

¼ cup full-fat mayonnaise

¼ cup chopped yellow onion

1 tablespoon dried parsley

¼ teaspoon salt

18 pieces sliced jalapeño from jar

2 tablespoons unsalted butter

1 Preheat oven to 350°F. Grease six cups of a muffin tin.

2 Combine all ingredients except the jalapeño slices and butter in a medium mixing bowl.

3 Evenly fill six muffin cups with the mixture, topping each with three jalapeño slices.

4 Bake 25 minutes. Serve warm with butter.

CHAPTER 9

DRINKS AND DESSERTS

Adulting. When I helped my husband research our last book, *DIRTY, LAZY, KETO Fast Food Guide: 10 Carbs or Less*, I was *astonished* to learn just how much sugar is hiding in America's favorite comfort drinks. Rest assured, you can still "get your drink on" while maintaining a DIRTY, LAZY, KETO lifestyle; this isn't prison! The whole point of this way of eating is *sustainability*. I don't know about your life, but mine includes a celebratory cocktail once in a while. In this chapter I will share some of my favorite hot, cold, and blended drinks.

It's not just sweet drinks that I love; I also crave sugary desserts. I've learned to work with my cravings for sweets by substituting sugar-free alternatives for sugar. *Notice I didn't say fat bombs!* I was recently quoted in *Reader's Digest* for coming out AGAINST the fat bomb. So controversial, I know!

> "I would rather the fat come from my 'booty' and not my Starbucks cup with HWC," I told the reporter. Yep, I sound THAT classy when sharing dieting advice to millions of readers.

When you're trying to achieve ketosis, or fat-burning mode, don't overfeed your metabolism with fat. In fact, it's counterproductive. My advice likely contradicts what you may have learned about keto before. I have an entirely different perspective on this topic.

While I completely support the role of sugar substitutes on DIRTY, LAZY, KETO, I recommend you enjoy them in recipes that don't call for an exorbitant amount of fat. The recipes I'm wagging my finger at, specifically, are the ones that call for cup after cup of heavy whipping cream. Those concoctions are not only likely to stall your weight loss, but might even take you to the dark side—*weight gain* (gasp!). Why would this happen? Fat is denser in calories than the other macronutrients, which means *a little goes a long way*. Yes, DIRTY, LAZY, KETO is fat-forward, but with a cautious recommendation to utilize fat for making healthy foods (like vegetables) taste better. Fat should be a lever, *not* a daily requirement that must be met. Instead of directly eating a spoonful of coconut oil, for example, use that oil to sauté asparagus.

While your physical sugar cravings wane, old habits and emotional triggers that scream for sugar often persist. Psychological hungers for sweets won't change overnight. In the meanwhile, I suggest "safe" sweet substitutes to keep on hand, which can help you get through moments when you MUST HAVE SOMETHING SWEET RIGHT NOW!

Yes, most of the sugar-free recipes or products I recommend contain artificial sweeteners or chemically processed ingredients.

Allowing and encouraging sugar-free substitutes is a key differentiator between Dirty Keto and Strict Keto.

The consumption of sugar substitutes is so controversial that it's almost a political stance, with mudslinging and screaming from both sides of the aisle. Before any rants ensue, let me be clear that DIRTY, LAZY, KETO supports the use of sugar substitutes to help you break the sugar-addicted cycle that led most of us to obesity. In all honesty, sometimes you have to choose the lesser of two evils.

Every product or recipe shared here is one that I personally used to successfully lose 140 pounds. In fact, I still enjoy these desserts, though admittedly with less frequency than when I first started.

PEPPERMINT PATTY HOT COCOA $ ✕

I adore all things chocolate, and when I'm feeling moody, I crave Peppermint Patty Hot Cocoa. Instead of reaching for candy, I created this simple, lightning-fast solution to meet my craving.

6 ounces hot water

1 tablespoon unsweetened cocoa powder

3 (1-gram) packets 0g net carb sweetener

½ teaspoon pure vanilla extract

1 tablespoon half and half

1 sugar-free peppermint hard candy

2 tablespoons canned whipped cream

1. Add all ingredients except whipped cream to a mug and stir until blended. Use an immersion blender if feeling fancy; otherwise, stirring by hand will do the job just fine.

2. Top with the whipped cream.

NET CARBS	
6G	

SERVES 1	

PER SERVING:	
CALORIES	67
FAT	4G
PROTEIN	2G
SODIUM	7MG
FIBER	2G
CARBOHYDRATES	10G
SUGAR	2G
SUGAR ALCOHOL	2G

TIME	
PREP TIME:	2 MIN
COOK TIME:	0 MIN

TIPS & OPTIONS

Top Peppermint Patty Hot Cocoa with sugar-free chocolate chips if you are in an especially chocolaty mood. If you have trouble preventing yourself from squirting whipped cream into your mouth, feel free to omit that ingredient!

In lieu of half and half, you may use ½ tablespoon heavy cream.

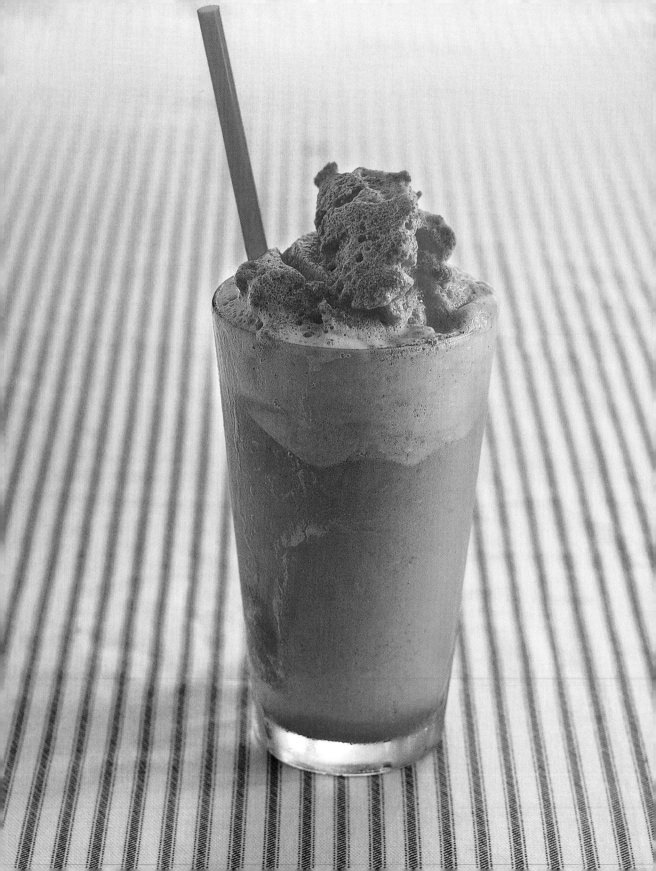

TACO BELL STRAWBERRY FREEZE $ ✕ 🍃 ◣

This past summer, I enjoyed one of these almost every day! This might stem from my "extreme" personality, but I've noticed that when I find a food that I like, I tend to get obsessed with it for a while. This dessert is low impact (only 1g net carbs), quick to make, and will instantly cure a raging sweet tooth. You may have already stumbled upon a variation of this recipe. Be forewarned, however, if you see it calls for **cup after cup** of heavy whipping cream (HWC). I urge you pass on those experiments for weight gain! Trust me, only a splash of dairy fat is what you need to make this recipe a winner.

2 cups ice

1 (9-gram) box strawberry sugar-free Jell-O gelatin

1 cup sugar-free flavored seltzer water (any flavor)

2 tablespoons half and half

Add all ingredients to a blender and pulse until ice is smooth (like a Frosty). Serve immediately.

NET CARBS	
1G	

SERVES 1	
PER SERVING:	
CALORIES	75
FAT	3G
PROTEIN	4G
SODIUM	210MG
FIBER	0G
CARBOHYDRATES	1G
SUGAR	1G

TIME	
PREP TIME:	3 MIN
COOK TIME:	0 MIN

◀◀ TIPS & OPTIONS

The varieties of this dessert are ENDLESS! Don't be afraid to experiment with any flavor of diet soda in lieu of seltzer water. You may want to let the soda pop "fizzle" out a bit before adding to the blender, however—you don't want an explosion on your hands (*which has actually happened to me, by the way*).

MCDONALD'S VANILLA SHAKE $

NET CARBS

4G

SERVES 1

PER SERVING:

CALORIES	176
FAT	6G
PROTEIN	23G
SODIUM	157MG
FIBER	1G
CARBOHYDRATES	5G
SUGAR	3G

TIME

PREP TIME:	3 MIN
COOK TIME:	0 MIN

TIPS & OPTIONS »

Make this drink a strawberry shake by substituting vanilla protein powder for berry-flavored protein powder. Add a few strawberries (fresh or frozen) to the blender and voilà! You'll have a pretty pink-colored strawberry shake.

Take your dirty keto to the extreme and experiment by adding a drop of inexpensive artificial flavors to your milkshake (so far, I've tried cake batter, cheesecake, red velvet, and lemon). Flavors can be purchased in the baking section at several big-box stores or ordered online.

Whenever I was sick as a child (which was often since my dad smoked inside our home), my mom would take me to McDonald's for a vanilla milkshake. Now that I'm an adult, I sneeze just once and have a Pavlovian response to drive toward the Golden Arches.

2 tablespoons canned whipped cream, divided

2 cups ice

3 tablespoons half and half

2 cups water

1 teaspoon pure vanilla extract

6 (1-gram) packets 0g net carb sweetener

1 (1-ounce) scoop 0g net carb vanilla protein powder

1 In a small blender, pulse 1 tablespoon whipped cream and all remaining ingredients until it reaches desired consistency.

2 Pour into a tall fancy glass and top with remaining tablespoon whipped cream. Enjoy!

REESE'S PEANUT BUTTER CUP SHAKE $

I panic every year on Halloween. It's not the costumes that scare me—it's the miniature-sized Reese's Peanut Butter Cups calling my name from the candy bowl. Knowing I have this shake in my arsenal helps keep my DLK armor strong.

2 cups ice

2 tablespoons no-sugar-added almond butter

2 cups water

6 (1-gram) packets 0g net carb sweetener

1 (1-ounce) scoop 0g net carb chocolate protein powder

⅛ teaspoon salt

1 tablespoon unsweetened cocoa powder, divided

2 tablespoons canned whipped cream

1 To a blender add all ingredients except whipped cream and a dash cocoa powder. Process until smooth.

2 Pour into a tall fancy glass and top with whipped cream. Sprinkle remaining cocoa powder on top and serve with a straw.

NET CARBS
5G

SERVES 1

PER SERVING:

CALORIES	314
FAT	18G
PROTEIN	30G
SODIUM	432MG
FIBER	6G
CARBOHYDRATES	11G
SUGAR	2G

TIME

PREP TIME:	3 MIN
COOK TIME:	0 MIN

TIPS & OPTIONS

Instead of water, try using leftover unsweetened coffee (both are zero carb).

Any nut butter will taste great in this concoction.

SECRET INGREDIENT CHOCOLATE PUDDING

TIPS & OPTIONS ≫

Use half and half or room-temperature coffee instead of water.

For flair, top your pudding with a dollop of real whipped cream from the can. If you're really trying to impress someone, decorate with a mint leaf and a raspberry!

My first "real" job was working at Wendy's fast-food restaurant, manning the salad bar. While I hated cleaning the sneeze guard (who invented that name?), I loved refilling the canned chocolate pudding. This recipe is my attempt to re-create that salad bar pudding.

2 tablespoons unsweetened cocoa powder

1 medium avocado, peeled, pitted, and chopped

8–10 drops liquid 0g net carb sweetener

½ teaspoon pure vanilla extract

1 medium ice cube

¼ cup water

⅛ teaspoon salt

1   In a small blender on high speed, combine all ingredients except salt.

2   Salt before serving, which interestingly enough, brings out chocolate flavor.

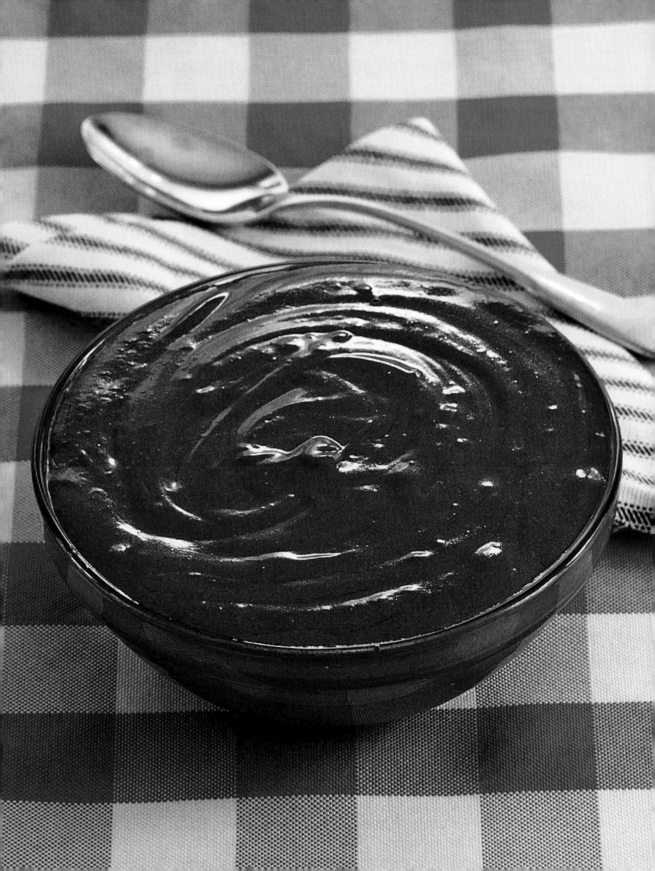

HIGH-ENERGY COCKTAIL HOUR

TIPS & OPTIONS

Other sugar-free mixer ideas are sugar-free flavored or unflavored seltzer water, sugar-free soda, mineral water, or plain water with a water flavor packet.

Of course, any unflavored hard alcohol will have exactly the same net carb count—ZERO!—and can be substituted to your tastes.

*Coming in second place behind questions about Bulletproof coffee is the nervously asked burning question: **Can I drink alcohol?** The quick answer is YES! This isn't prison, after all. You can certainly enjoy your low-carb cocktail providing your lowered inhibitions don't lead you astray at the snack bar.*

1 cup ice
1 (8-ounce) zero-carb energy drink
1 shot unflavored vodka
1 slice lime

In a fancy glass, mix ice, energy drink, and vodka. Garnish with lime. Cheers!

CINNAMON CHURROS $ ✕ 🌿

Even though these keto Cinnamon Churros may not look exactly like the churros you know, you'll appreciate how similarly they mimic the taste of the original.

Churros
⅔ cup unblanched almond flour

¼ cup coconut flour

1 tablespoon flaxseed meal

1 teaspoon xanthan gum

1 cup water

¼ cup unsalted butter

2 tablespoons 0g net carb sweetener

¼ teaspoon salt

2 large eggs, lightly beaten

1 teaspoon pure vanilla extract

Garnish
1 tablespoon unsalted butter, melted

2 teaspoons ground cinnamon

¼ cup 0g net carb sweetener

NET CARBS
2G

SERVES 12

PER SERVING:

CALORIES	106
FAT	9G
PROTEIN	3G
SODIUM	64MG
FIBER	2G
CARBOHYDRATES	4G
SUGAR	1G

TIME	
PREP TIME:	25 MIN
COOK TIME:	30 MIN

1. Preheat oven to 350°F. Line a large baking sheet with parchment paper.

2. In a medium bowl, whisk together almond flour, coconut flour, flaxseed meal, and xanthan gum.

3. In a medium pot over medium heat, heat water almost to a boil and mix in ¼ cup butter, 2 tablespoons sweetener, and ¼ teaspoon salt until butter is melted and well blended. Add flour mix and keep stirring until a ball is formed.

4. Return dough to bowl and let cool for 5 minutes. Mix eggs and vanilla in with dough.

5. Let dough cool to room temperature, 10–15 minutes. Transfer dough into a pastry piping bag with star tip. Make twelve churros and place on baking sheet.

6. Bake 15–20 minutes until deep golden.

7. Remove from oven and brush with butter. Garnish with cinnamon and sweetener. Serve warm.

≪ TIPS & OPTIONS

Instead of messing around with cumbersome pastry bags, I substitute a disposable Ziploc bag. The freezer-type bag has the strongest seams and won't rip when squeezing out the pastry dough. Cut a corner off the Ziploc bag to make a hole of the proper width (approximately ⅜"), fill with the dough, and gently squeeze out the churro. To keep it simple, you can just make a round churro and skip the star pastry tip. This trick makes cleanup a breeze!

You can easily alter this recipe to six servings by only making six churros that are twice the length of the original; these churros are low-carb enough to safely splurge on.

HAWAIIAN SHAVED ICE $ ◎ ✕ 🌱 🥣

TIPS & OPTIONS 》》

Adults have the option of adding a little "somethin' somethin'" to their Hawaiian Shaved Ice. A splash (or two) of unflavored rum adds zero carbs, but definitely increases the fun factor!

Try to get the funnel-shaped paper cups to increase the fun factor.

These are zero carb, so go nuts and double the recipe to make some extra-large and extra-fun Hawaiian Shaved Ice!

*We are lucky to have visited "the islands" many times over the years. Hawaiian Shaved Ice is a popular and colorful dessert (reminiscent of the snow cone from my childhood). This simple, yet delicious dessert will stop you dead in your tracks if you try to eat too much too quickly—**can you say "ice cream headache"**? Make this treat at home with the help of flavored sugar-free syrups. They come in every flavor, from watermelon to lemon to pineapple—all sugar-free! Check your local dollar store, discount grocery store, or even online to find your favorite flavor.*

4 cups crushed ice

8 tablespoons sugar-free, zero carb tropical-flavored syrup (flavors of your choosing)

1 Blend ice in a blender to the desired consistency and scoop evenly into four cups.

2 Top each with 2 tablespoons sugar-free flavoring (preferably in varying colors).

YELLOW SNOW SORBET $ ◉ ✗ ✐ ▼

*I might be a rare bird, but I prefer lemon over chocolate-flavored desserts any day. Since my days of lemon meringue pie are behind me, I am happy to make this sugar-free icy alternative. Yellow Snow Sorbet is fancy enough to serve to guests (**but don't tell them the awful name!**). Unless you're willing to risk a painful ice cream headache, the built-in portion control of a frozen dessert will stop you from eating too much.*

½ cup 0g net carb sweetener

4 cups water

¾ cup lemon juice, from concentrate

1   In a medium saucepan over medium heat, mix sweetener into hot water. Stir 5 minutes until all sweetener is dissolved.

2   Stir in lemon juice.

3   Remove from flame and let cool for 5 minutes.

4   Transfer mixture to a 9" × 5" × 2½" loaf pan. Place in freezer for 1½ hours.

5   Remove from freezer and whisk thoroughly. Return to the freezer and whisk every ½ hour for 3–4 more hours until desired consistency is reached.

6   Serve in four festive glasses.

NET CARBS
3G

SERVES 4

PER SERVING:

CALORIES	10
FAT	0G
PROTEIN	0G
SODIUM	0MG
FIBER	0G
CARBOHYDRATES	3G
SUGAR	1G

TIME

PREP TIME:	5 MIN
COOK TIME:	5 MIN

◀◀ TIPS & OPTIONS

For added drama and flair, serve this dessert inside hollowed-out lemons.

To save time, try this shortcut: Use a commercial blender to smooth out the cooled lemon mixture with cups of ice.

Want to make an even lower net carb version? Skip the natural juices and substitute sugar-free lemonade water flavor packets instead.

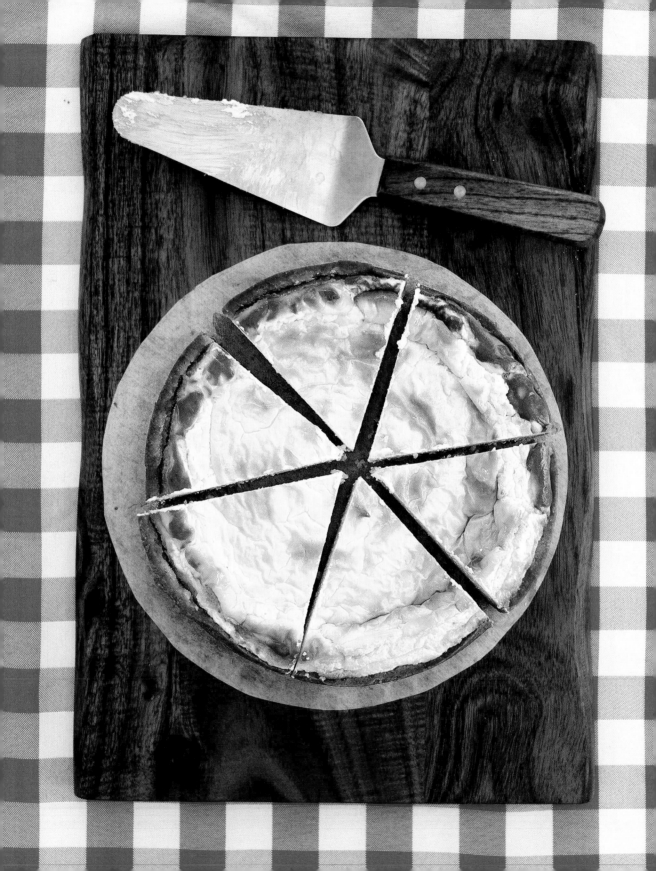

BIRTHDAY CHEESECAKE

*Birthday Cheesecake looks and tastes so close to the real thing that no one will ever be able to tell it's not! When I make this dessert, I will obsess over it so much that I end up eating slices at breakfast, lunch, and dinner, **one meal after the next**, until it's all gone. Clearly, I love sweets! Even though Birthday Cheesecake is low in net carbs, I have to limit how often I have desserts like this available in my home. It's just too tempting for me! Know thyself, friends. This recipe technically serves sixteen, but that almost makes me laugh out loud. I won't share it with anyone!*

Crust
2 cups blanched almond flour

⅓ cup unsalted butter, melted

3 tablespoons 0g net carb sweetener

1 teaspoon pure vanilla extract

Cheesecake Filling
32 ounces full-fat cream cheese, softened

¾ cup full-fat sour cream

1¼ cups 0g net carb sweetener

3 large eggs, room temperature

1 tablespoon lemon juice

1½ teaspoons pure vanilla extract

NET CARBS	
7G	
SERVES 16	
PER SERVING:	
CALORIES	343
FAT	28G
PROTEIN	9G
SODIUM	225MG
FIBER	1G
CARBOHYDRATES	8G
SUGAR	3G

TIME	
PREP TIME:	30 MIN
COOK TIME:	1 HR 15 MIN

1 Preheat oven to 350°F.

2 Generously grease the sides of a 9" springform pan. Cut some parchment paper to line the bottom and grease it as well.

3 For the crust, mix the almond flour, melted butter, sweetener, and vanilla in a medium bowl. Finished product will be dry. Spread and pack crust evenly onto bottom of the pan. Bake crust 10–15 minutes or until golden brown.

4 Using an electric mixer, in a large bowl, beat softened cream cheese, sour cream, and sweetener on low speed while ensuring there are not too many bubbles in the mix. Beat eggs in one at a time. Stop and scrape bowl periodically to ensure all ingredients completely mix. Beat in lemon juice and vanilla extract.

5 Pour batter on top of cooked crust and level the top. Bake 50–60 minutes until center is almost set.

6 Remove from oven. Use a sharp knife to cut around edge. Let cool 10 minutes. Refrigerate in pan 4 hours. Release from the pan when ready to serve.

TIPS & OPTIONS

If desired, you can top with fresh berries and real whipped cream from the can.

You can skip the crust to reduce the carb count by 2g net carbs per serving.

Over the years, I have experimented with different ingredients for the crust: crushed pretzels (*gasp!*), crushed pecans, and unsweetened shredded coconut are fun ingredients to experiment with.

For cheesecake custard variety, experiment by creating new cheesecake flavors: adding additional strawberry sugar-free powdered Jell-O, or unsweetened cocoa powder.

PISTACHIO FLUFFER-NUTTER $ ✕ 🌱

NET CARBS

6G

SERVES 6

PER SERVING:

CALORIES	214
FAT	18G
PROTEIN	3G
SODIUM	370MG
FIBER	0G
CARBOHYDRATES	6G
SUGAR	2G

TIME

PREP TIME:	5 MIN
COOK TIME:	0 MIN

TIPS & OPTIONS　》》

Add chopped nuts, fruit, or berries as toppings.

At my house, Fluffer-Nutter never makes it out of the mixing bowl. I lick 100 percent of the batter from the mixing bowl using a spatula. For that reason, I don't make this very often myself! My kind daughter, on the other hand, will make this recipe for me while I'm **sitting on my hands** *in another room. When it's served to me (by someone else) in a single portion, I am able to enjoy the dessert* **like a normal person** *and stop myself from eating the entire bowl.*

8 ounces full-fat cream cheese, softened

1 teaspoon pure vanilla extract

⅛ teaspoon salt

1 (1-ounce) package sugar-free pistachio-flavored instant pudding

¼ cup 0g net carb sweetener

½ cup heavy whipping cream

1   In a medium mixing bowl with electric beaters at slow speed to start, combine cream cheese, vanilla, salt, pudding, and sweetener.

2   Mix thoroughly at medium speed, stopping periodically to scrape bowl and beaters to ensure complete mixing.

3   Start mixer again at medium to high speed and slowly add heavy whipping cream until the mixture becomes a foam. Continue until foam has sturdy peaks.

4   Serve immediately or cover and refrigerate.

5   Pudding will keep three to four days if properly refrigerated.

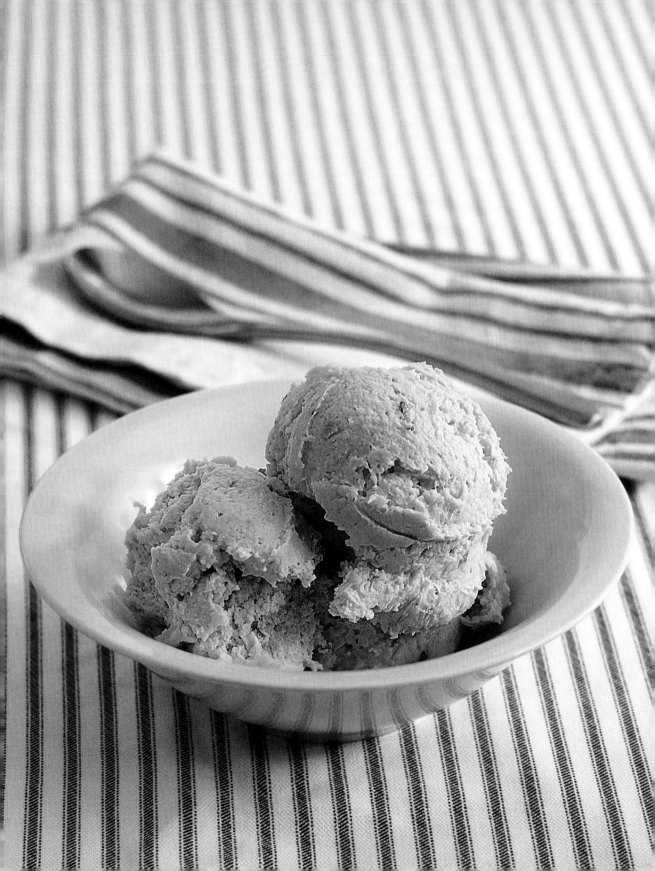

CHILLED PEANUT BUTTER BLOSSOMS

$ ◎ ✕ 🌱

TIPS & OPTIONS ≫

I sometimes substitute zero carb chocolate protein powder for coconut flour.

If I'm feeling fancy, I might sprinkle the balls with (or roll them in) additional sugar-free sweetener prior to topping with a chocolate chip. This helps make the cookie look more like the peanut blossoms that I grew up with.

Since there is no oven involved, Chilled Peanut Butter Blossoms is a recipe that even your kids can make. This recipe is my best substitute for the Hershey's Kiss cookies I used to make every year during the holidays. The cookies freeze well when layered with wax paper. (But who has extra to freeze?) **Not me!**

2 cups no-sugar-added peanut butter

½ cup 0g net carb sweetener

¾ cup coconut flour

1 teaspoon water

24 sugar-free chocolate chips, approximately ¼ cup

1 Line a baking sheet with parchment paper.

2 Place all ingredients in a large mixing bowl. Mix well.

3 Form twenty-four small balls about ¾" in diameter with batter and place on baking sheet. Push one sugar-free chocolate chip onto each ball.

4 Refrigerate 30 minutes until firm.

DEBAUCHERY CHOCOLATE BROWNIES

*Trust me, you will bookmark this page. This simple recipe will be one of your go-to desserts. It tastes **just like the real thing**, and it's quick and easy to make.*

¾ cup unsalted butter, softened

3 large eggs

¾ cup Carbquik, divided

1 cup powdered 0g net carb sweetener

½ cup finely chopped pecans

1 cup Lily's sugar-free chocolate chips

¾ cup unsweetened cocoa powder

½ teaspoon salt

1 Preheat oven to 325°F. Grease and "flour" an 8" × 8" pan (using 1 tablespoon Carbquik).

2 In a large bowl, beat butter with eggs.

3 In a medium bowl, combine the dry ingredients and add to the large bowl. Mix in the remaining ingredients to form batter.

4 Spread mixture into pan and bake 30 minutes. Use a toothpick to tell if it's done by poking it into center—it should come out clean.

5 Cut into sixteen portions and serve while still warm.

NET CARBS

8G

SERVES 16

PER SERVING:

CALORIES	184
FAT	17G
PROTEIN	4G
SODIUM	117MG
FIBER	8G
CARBOHYDRATES	23G
SUGAR	0G
SUGAR ALCOHOL	7G

TIME

PREP TIME:	10 MIN
COOK TIME:	30 MIN

TIPS & OPTIONS

Feel free to skip the nuts in this recipe.

Make clean cuts to your brownie squares by cutting squares with a plastic knife.

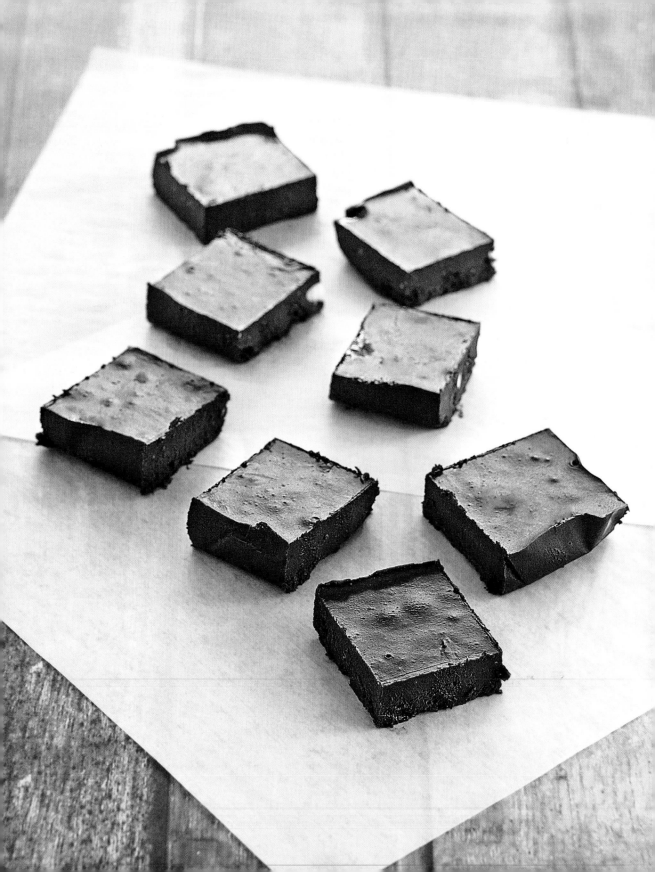

F-U-D-G-E $ ◉ ✕ ❀

When my kids were little, we as adults often spoke in code. Since I didn't know pig Latin, I would spell out forbidden words. My son picked up on this one really quickly, F-U-D-G-E! Five simple ingredients are all it takes to build this wondrous creation. Since I struggle with portion control around sweets (that's a fancy way of saying that I will make myself sick by eating the entire pan at once), I freeze individual portions of the fudge using snack-sized Ziploc bags.

½ cup no-sugar-added peanut butter

¼ cup coconut oil

3 tablespoons unsweetened cocoa powder

3 tablespoons 0g net carb sweetener

½ teaspoon pure vanilla extract

1 Add all the ingredients to a large bowl and mix well.

2 Transfer mixture into a 4" × 8" loaf pan lined with parchment paper or a similar-sized silicon mold.

3 Freeze 30 minutes (until firm).

4 Cut fudge into eight pieces and return to freezer.

NET CARBS

1G

SERVES 8

PER SERVING:

CALORIES	163
FAT	15G
PROTEIN	4G
SODIUM	0MG
FIBER	2G
CARBOHYDRATES	3G
SUGAR	1G

TIME

PREP TIME:	10 MIN
COOK TIME:	0 MIN

≪ TIPS & OPTIONS

Make your fudge even more delicious by topping it with peanuts, sliced almonds, crushed walnuts, sugar-free chocolate chips, or shredded unsweetened coconut.

Keep your fudge in the freezer and it will last for weeks. It won't freeze since it is mostly oil and there is very little water that can freeze.

AFTER-DINNER PARFAIT $ ◉ ✕ 🌱 🥣

NET CARBS	
2G	

SERVES 4

PER SERVING:

CALORIES	122
FAT	10G
PROTEIN	3G
SODIUM	159MG
FIBER	0G
CARBOHYDRATES	2G
SUGAR	1G

TIME

PREP TIME:	10 MIN
COOK TIME:	0 MIN

TIPS & OPTIONS ≫

When making your Jell-O, try substituting cold flavored, sugar-free seltzer water for the 1 cup of cold tap water.

Instead of full-fat cream cheese, try substituting full-fat sour cream. It gives the dessert a sweet-and-sour tanginess!

Want to skip a step? Sometimes I purchase premade sugar-free Jell-O cups and stir in a spoonful of desired cream (sour cream or cream cheese).

Stemming from a desire to break a weight loss stall, I developed a personal rule early in my weight loss journey to "cold stop" all eating after I finished my dinner. Don't laugh, but as a result of this arbitrary rule, I often find myself sitting alone at the kitchen table, long after my family finishes eating. I never want to leave the table, as getting up signifies that my "eating window" is over for the day! Enjoying an After-Dinner Parfait helps me top off my meal with something sweet before entering a period of Intermittent Fasting.

1 small (9-gram) package sugar-free Jell-O, any flavor

1 cup boiling water

1 cup cold water

4 ounces full-fat cream cheese, softened

2 tablespoons canned whipped cream

1 tablespoon crushed salty peanuts

1   In a medium bowl, add Jell-O to boiling water. Stir in cold water until mixture starts to thicken, 2–3 minutes. Refrigerate until firm, about 30 minutes.

2   Using a mixer in a medium mixing bowl, beat softened cream cheese until smooth. Going slowly at first, combine firm Jell-O with cream cheese. Gradually increase speed until desired consistency is reached.

3   Scoop into serving bowls and top with whipped cream and dusting of crushed peanuts.

CINNAMON TOAST CRUNCH NUTS

*Because nuts are so easy to overeat, I am hesitant to share my Cinnamon Toast Crunch Nuts recipe with you. I have trouble stopping myself after eating just one serving. While I normally double or triple most recipes (to save some for later), that strategy is **definitely not** recommended here. In fact, I've even burned my mouth (NUMEROUS TIMES) while impatiently neglecting to allow the nuts in this recipe to sufficiently cool. In an ideal world, I would sprinkle this finished product on top of a light summer salad with goat cheese and strawberries. But that has yet to happen! I eat them as soon as they are ready.*

1 tablespoon unsalted butter, softened

¼ cup pecan halves

¼ teaspoon pure vanilla extract

4 tablespoons 0g net carb sweetener

⅛ teaspoon ground cinnamon

1   In a small saucepan over low heat, toss all ingredients starting with the butter until well coated and toasted (up to 5 minutes).

2   Spread out and let cool on wax or parchment paper to prevent sticking together.

NET CARBS	
1G	
SERVES 1	
PER SERVING:	
CALORIES	275
FAT	28G
PROTEIN	2G
SODIUM	1MG
FIBER	3G
CARBOHYDRATES	4G
SUGAR	1G

TIME	
PREP TIME:	1 MIN
COOK TIME:	5 MIN

TIPS & OPTIONS

Don't like pecans? Substitute your favorite low-carb nut.

If you prefer more of a pecan brittle, add 4 teaspoons monk fruit sweetener (0g net carbs per serving) to the rest of the ingredients in the saucepan. Pour remaining monk fruit liquid over your pecans on the wax paper. The liquid will dry and crumble similar to peanut brittle.

Drizzle melted sugar-free chocolate or sprinkle toasted coconut over your finished nuts to make the dessert even more seductive.

MAHALO COCONUT MACAROONS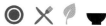

NET CARBS

1G

SERVES 24

PER SERVING:

CALORIES	47
FAT	4G
PROTEIN	1G
SODIUM	9MG
FIBER	1G
CARBOHYDRATES	2G
SUGAR	1G

TIME

PREP TIME:	10 MIN
COOK TIME:	12 MIN

TIPS & OPTIONS

Drizzle melted sugar-free chocolate onto macaroons for added decadence.

Feel free to double the size of the balls and make 12 serving (all macronutrients will be doubled).

*I crack up hearing criticism about keto desserts. Folks will complain that sugar-free desserts don't taste as good as normal desserts made with real sugar. **Well, duh!** That shouldn't be surprising. Of course, sugar-free desserts taste different because they **lack…you guessed it, SUGAR!** Sugar substitutes taste different to each individual person. It's like how some people think cilantro tastes like soap. Find one that is "most tolerable" to you and stick with it. That's the best I can do.*

4 large egg whites

3 tablespoons 0g net carb sweetener

2 cups unsweetened shredded coconut

1 teaspoon pure vanilla extract

1 Preheat oven to 350°F. Line a baking sheet with parchment paper.

2 In a medium bowl, whisk egg whites, then add sweetener.

3 Combine egg white mixture with shredded coconut and vanilla.

4 Spoon twenty-four small balls (approximately ¾") onto baking sheet.

5 Cook 10–12 minutes or until golden brown.

6 Remove from oven and serve warm.

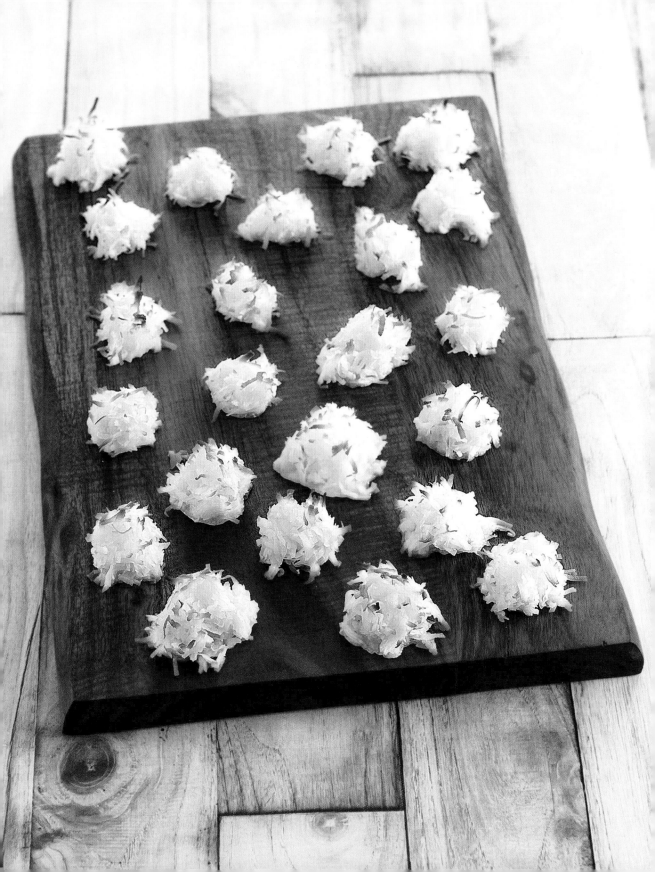

ADDITIONAL RESOURCES

KEEP TALKIN' DIRTY TO ME

To help support my readers, I host several *Facebook* groups of varying levels of support. Available 24/7, you will find like-minded DIRTY, LAZY, KETO followers to answer your questions and provide encouragement. The first group started with only my best friend and my husband, but has since blossomed to the size of a metropolis in just months. Join for free at www.facebook.com/groups/dirtylazyketo.

Be forewarned…with so many members, this group can sometimes be the Keto Wild West!

If a smaller, more private, intimate support group would better meet your needs, I also host a limited enrollment, subscription-based Premium group for women only, where I'm directly involved in every post: www.facebook.com/groups/DIRTYLAZYKETO.Premium/.

If you need additional sass and support, look no further than *DIRTY, LAZY, KETO: Get Started Losing Weight While Breaking the Rules* by Stephanie Laska and *DIRTY, LAZY, KETO Fast Food Guide: 10 Carbs or Less* by William Laska and Stephanie Laska.

In case you'd like to read more about the science behind the keto diet, I encourage you to learn from the anti-sugar guru himself, Gary Taubes. I highly recommend his books, *Why We Get Fat: And What to Do about It*; *Good Calories, Bad Calories*; and

The Case Against Sugar. Next, check out Dr. Jason Fung's *The Obesity Code* to learn more about the science behind intermittent fasting and why calorie-restrictive diets ultimately backfire.

If you want to work on establishing healthier habits, look no further than my favorite author, Gretchen Rubin. Whether you listen to her *Happier* podcast or read *The Four Tendencies*, you are sure to walk away with a clearer understanding of your own personality. She helped me learn how to harness my personality type to create more desirable eating and exercise habits.

To receive *free* ongoing articles and tips to help you in your weight loss journey, register your email at DirtyLazyKeto.com.

For continued social media updates, interact with DIRTY, LAZY, KETO:

+ *Facebook*: @DIRTYLAZYKETO
+ *Instagram*: @140Lost and @DIRTYLAZYKETO
+ *Pinterest*: @DIRTYLAZYKETO
+ *Twitter*: @140Lost
+ *YouTube*: http://bit.ly/DLKYouTube
+ Podcast? Listen to the *DIRTY, LAZY, Girl* Podcast on Apple Podcasts, Spotify, or Google Podcasts

For additional resources, visit the author's website: DirtyLazyKeto.com.

#KETOON! MARCHING ORDERS

Hold your head up high, fellow ketonian! You may be marching to a unique drum with this lifestyle, but I assure you it is a path toward long-lasting success. DIRTY, LAZY, KETO is not a diet; *it's a way of life.*

Thank you for coming on this journey with *The DIRTY, LAZY, KETO Cookbook*. Pay it forward! Help others discover this lifestyle by leaving an honest review wherever you shop for books.

TERMS FOR DIRTY, LAZY, KETO

As a courtesy, I've included a glossary of commonly used keto terms. Keep in mind that my definition of the term might be different from what you have heard before.

CALORIES

Calories are the units of heat food provides to the body. There are no "good" or "bad" calories. You've got to let this one go, people! Calories are just an innocent unit of measurement, like a cup or a gallon. Our bodies *require* calories to survive. With DIRTY, LAZY, KETO, calories are not the focus (instead, net carbs are). The 1980s are over, my friends, and counting only calories of low-fat foods is just as passé as leg warmers.

CARBOHYDRATES (CARBS)

Carbohydrates (or "Carbs" for short) are sugars, starches, and fibers found in fruits, grains, vegetables, and milk products. Foods high in carbs include bread, pasta, beans, potatoes, rice, and cereals. In general, packaged or processed foods in your pantry are likely high in carb content. Carbs contain four calories per gram. To further break down this macro group, I reclassified carbs into two unique subcategories:

+ Slow-Burning Carbs (my own made-up term) have a high fiber content and lower glycemic index. They are less likely to cause a spike in blood sugar. Slow-burning carbs are more desirable (in my opinion) as they keep you feeling full for longer. They offer your body overall better health benefits when compared to fast-burning carbs. Examples include nonstarchy, high-fiber vegetables like celery and broccoli. *Slow-burning carbs are your weight loss best friends!* They are more helpful for your well-being than simple, fast-burning carbs in maintaining steady blood sugar levels. Slow-burning carbs prevent a backlash of sugar cravings.

+ Fast-Burning Carbs (again, not a scientific phrase, just my own jargon) are simple sugars that quickly release glucose into the bloodstream. These include processed carbohydrates like breads, cereals, sugars, high-sugar fruits, and some starchy veg-etables. Examples include candy, soda, pasta, potatoes, popcorn, tortillas, and bananas. This is the category of foods that has caused me so much trouble!

COUNTING MACROS

Instead of counting calories, many keto dieters track their intake of macronutrients (proteins, fats, and carbohydrates). You hear the phrase "counting macros" often in keto-land. Dieters might have a goal or a limit for each category, or a specific ratio to achieve each day with their eating choices. If needed for accuracy and moti-vation, apps and food calculators can be used to track daily food choices. While everyone goes about this in slightly different ways, note that the only macro I ever counted was the carbohydrate.

DIRTY KETO

Dirty Keto includes eating whatever foods you choose within your macro goals or limits (which are different for everyone). Dirty Keto followers have a reputation (which may or may not be true) for including keto junk food in their diet (no judgment!). For example, if you want to eat a hot dog, then have at it, sister. This is your body, and only you can decide what to eat or drink. Dirty Keto means you can play dirty and don't have to follow specific rules about your eating (other than the "big picture" of counting macros). Artificial sweeteners and low-carb substitutes are fair game. Dirty Keto followers don't limit their food or beverage choices, and might even be spotted drinking a Diet Coke (Oh, the horror!).

DIRTY AND LAZY KETO

Dirty and Lazy Keto dieters are a modern hybrid that reap even more benefits of losing weight on a keto diet, but without limitations of food choices or the obligation of counting every macro. They are open to the idea of artificial sweeteners (the aspartame in Diet Coke or Splenda, for example) and packaged foods (protein bars, low-carb tortillas) as part of their diet as long as they don't cause them to exceed their daily net carb limit. Dirty and Lazy Keto followers count only the carbs they eat each day. *I am the superhero of this category!*

FATS

Fats are the densest form of energy, providing nine calories per gram. The most obvious example of fats is oil (olive, coconut, sesame, canola, vegetable, and so on). Less clear examples of fats are dairy foods like cream, butter, or cheese. Some fats have a better reputation than others. Think about how the media portrays eggs, full-fat mayonnaise, Alfredo sauce, or chicken skin. While all fattening, everyone has strong opinions about whether these foods should be part of your diet. I've been told to even avoid salmon, nuts, and avocado for fear of eating too much fat. No matter what the quality of the source, fat is fat is fat.

FAT BOMBS

Fat bombs are low-carb, high-fat desserts that are usually artificially sweetened.

KETO

Keto is simply a shortened word for ketogenic. It sounds a bit sexier and less medical, so let's go with that.

KETOGENIC DIET

A ketogenic diet consists of eating a diet of foods that are low in carbohydrates, moderate in protein, and higher in fat, with the goal of going into ketosis.

KETONES

Ketones are acids. Ketones occur when fat is breaking down. Ketones are often found in the blood and urine during weight loss.

KETONE URINE TESTING STRIPS

Ketone urine testing strips are just what you might expect. They are little strips of paper that, when dipped in your urine, will identify if your body has reached ketosis, or weight loss mode. I have never used a ketone urine testing strip in my life, but I wanted to let you know about their availability. I suspect just getting on the scale might be cheaper than buying these (*and less messy—just sayin'*).

KETOSIS

Ketosis occurs when the body burns ketones from the liver as the main energy source for the body (as opposed to using glucose as the energy source derived from carbs). Ketosis is often an indicator (but not a requirement) of weight loss.

LAZY KETO

Lazy Keto followers count only carb intake, and do not track their consumption of fat grams or grams of protein. Lazy Keto does *not* mean unwilling to work hard for weight loss. This term refers to the method of counting a single macro in keto—the carb—not a relaxed lifestyle/lack of energy.

LCHF

LCHF is a diet that consists of eating Low-Carbohydrate, High-Fat foods without the goal of ketosis. You may be totally shocked to learn that some skinny folks eat LCHF for reasons other than weight loss! Benefits of eating LCHF might include a reduction of inflammation, decreased joint pain, increased energy, or weight loss maintenance.

MACRONUTRIENTS (MACROS)

There are three macronutrients: carbohydrates, proteins, and fats. All macronutrients must be obtained through foods in the diet as the body cannot produce them. Macronutrients are necessary for fuel. There are no "good" macros or "bad" macros (though one of them is definitely my favorite—*ahhh, carbs*). Each macro fulfills vital roles with nutrition and your health. All macros contain calories, but at different densities.

NET CARBS

Net carbs are the unit of measurement tracked in DIRTY, LAZY, KETO. When looking at a nutrition label, net carbs are calculated by subtracting all fiber grams and sugar alcohol grams from the listed amount of carbohydrates. Net carbs are the carbs left over in this mathematical equation. (Sugar, as a side note, is *not* subtracted—*sorry!*)

PROTEIN

Protein has four calories per gram. Proteins take longer to digest since they are long-chain amino acids. Protein is largely found in meats, dairy, eggs, soy, nuts, and seafood.

STRICT KETO

Strict Keto can go several ways. There are multiple factions within Strict Keto:

+ *Dirty Strict Keto* followers are sometimes dirty with their ingredient choices, but still identify as strict because they prefer to count all of their macros (fat, protein, carbs, and maybe even calories). They will count, and potentially enjoy, artificial sweeteners, grain-based fillers, chemical additives, and sugar substitutes.
+ *Bi-Strict Keto* followers lurk in the middle ground between Strict and Dirty. Bi-Strict Keto dieters go back and forth, becoming stricter (if needed) to break a weight loss stall. Or, they might "eat clean" most of the time, but allow for little treats like a Diet Coke or low-carb ice cream once in a while. While their belief system is different than mine, I admire how Bi-Strict Keto dieters are doing what works for them. I recognize my way isn't the only way; flexibility and style are important.
+ *Keto Purists* are the most extreme of all keto followers; they completely avoid artificial or chemically processed foods, and may demand absolute organic, natural ingredients. As with every faction, there may be those who believe their clean eating lifestyle makes them better than everyone else. Keto police jump out at you on social media because of their high-and-mighty attitude. Here, even the tiniest of carbs will be called

out and punished with their loud voices: "STOP! Put that half and half down—it has 0.4g net carbs per serving!" Keto Purists count carbs from just a splash of soy sauce or a sugar-free cough drop. Often, because they don't have enough to do already (*sarcasm*), Keto Purists document calories in addition to strategically calculating ongoing macro goals and limits.

If you are still not sure what keto camp you fall into, try taking the free short quiz I created on my website: https://dirtylazyketo.com/quiz.

US/METRIC CONVERSION CHARTS

VOLUME CONVERSIONS

US VOLUME MEASURE	METRIC EQUIVALENT
⅛ teaspoon	0.5 milliliter
¼ teaspoon	1 milliliter
½ teaspoon	2 milliliters
1 teaspoon	5 milliliters
½ tablespoon	7 milliliters
1 tablespoon (3 teaspoons)	15 milliliters
2 tablespoons (1 fluid ounce)	30 milliliters
¼ cup (4 tablespoons)	60 milliliters
⅓ cup	90 milliliters
½ cup (4 fluid ounces)	125 milliliters
⅔ cup	160 milliliters
¾ cup (6 fluid ounces)	180 milliliters
1 cup (16 tablespoons)	250 milliliters
1 pint (2 cups)	500 milliliters
1 quart (4 cups)	1 liter (about)

WEIGHT CONVERSIONS

US VOLUME MEASURE	METRIC EQUIVALENT
½ ounce	15 grams
1 ounce	30 grams
2 ounces	60 grams
3 ounces	85 grams
¼ pound (4 ounces)	115 grams
½ pound (8 ounces)	225 grams
¾ pound (12 ounces)	340 grams
1 pound (16 ounces)	454 grams

OVEN TEMPERATURE CONVERSIONS

DEGREES FAHRENHEIT	DEGREES CELSIUS
200 degrees F	95 degrees C
250 degrees F	120 degrees C
275 degrees F	135 degrees C
300 degrees F	150 degrees C
325 degrees F	160 degrees C
350 degrees F	180 degrees C
375 degrees F	190 degrees C
400 degrees F	205 degrees C
425 degrees F	220 degrees C
450 degrees F	230 degrees C

BAKING PAN SIZES

AMERICAN	METRIC
8 × 1½ inch round baking pan	20 × 4 cm cake tin
9 × 1½ inch round baking pan	23 × 3.5 cm cake tin
11 × 7 × 1½ inch baking pan	28 × 18 × 4 cm baking tin
13 × 9 × 2 inch baking pan	30 × 20 × 5 cm baking tin
2 quart rectangular baking dish	30 × 20 × 3 cm baking tin
15 × 10 × 2 inch baking pan	30 × 25 × 2 cm baking tin (Swiss roll tin)
9 inch pie plate	22 × 4 or 23 × 4 cm pie plate
7 or 8 inch springform pan	18 or 20 cm springform or loose bottom cake tin
9 × 5 × 3 inch loaf pan	23 × 13 × 7 cm or 2 lb narrow loaf or pate tin
1½ quart casserole	1.5 liter casserole
2 quart casserole	2 liter casserole

INDEX

Note: Page numbers in **bold** indicate recipe lists showing recipe category icons.

ABOUT THE AUTHORS

Stephanie Laska doesn't just talk the talk; she walks the walk. She is one of the few keto authors that has successfully lost half of her body weight (140 pounds!) and maintained that weight loss for six years and counting. Her sass and honest approach to keto dieting has been quoted in articles by *Reader's Digest, Playboy, Yahoo! News, First for Women* magazine, and *Costco Connection* magazine. Stephanie's story or image has been celebrated by *Muscle & Fitness: Hers*, the Big Sur International Marathon race guide, runDisney, and even a Groupon!

When she isn't writing about all things keto, Stephanie volunteers as a race Ambassador (San Francisco Marathon, Bay to Breakers) and Pacer to encourage more people to exercise. She has run a dozen marathons, most notably the New York City Marathon as a sponsored athlete from PowerBar. Not bad for a girl who ran her first mile (as in ever!) close to age forty.

Stephanie Laska, MEd, is also the author and creator of DIRTY, LAZY, KETO. Expect honesty and inspiration from your sassy girlfriend, Stephanie Laska—she shares the secret to losing weight and making this a permanent lifestyle in *DIRTY, LAZY, KETO: Get Started Losing Weight While Breaking the Rules*.

Additionally, Stephanie and her husband, William Laska, cowrote the extremely helpful support guide *DIRTY, LAZY, KETO Fast Food Guide: 10 Carbs or Less*, helping DIRTY, LAZY, KETO followers make the right decisions in the drive-thru.

Stephanie and Bill reside in sunny California. When they are not talking about their third child (DIRTY, LAZY, KETO), the Laskas enjoy running, traveling "on the cheap," and shopping at thrift stores.